Health Statistics: The Australian Experience and Opportunities

Health Statistics: The Australian Experience and Opportunities

Editor
Richard Madden

MDPI • Basel • Beijing • Wuhan • Barcelona • Belgrade • Manchester • Tokyo • Cluj • Tianjin

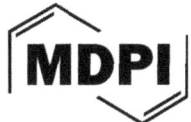

Editor
Richard Madden
Faculty of Medicine and Health,
The University of Sydney,
Sydney, NSW 2006, Australia

Editorial Office
MDPI
St. Alban-Anlage 66
4052 Basel, Switzerland

This is a reprint of articles from the Special Issue published online in the open access journal *International Journal of Environmental Research and Public Health* (ISSN 1660-4601) (available at: https://www.mdpi.com/journal/ijerph/special_issues/Health_Statistics_Australian_Experience_Opportunities).

For citation purposes, cite each article independently as indicated on the article page online and as indicated below:

LastName, A.A.; LastName, B.B.; LastName, C.C. Article Title. *Journal Name* **Year**, *Volume Number*, Page Range.

ISBN 978-3-0365-4805-0 (Hbk)
ISBN 978-3-0365-4806-7 (PDF)

© 2022 by the authors. Articles in this book are Open Access and distributed under the Creative Commons Attribution (CC BY) license, which allows users to download, copy and build upon published articles, as long as the author and publisher are properly credited, which ensures maximum dissemination and a wider impact of our publications.

The book as a whole is distributed by MDPI under the terms and conditions of the Creative Commons license CC BY-NC-ND.

Contents

Preface to "Health Statistics: The Australian Experience and Opportunities" vii

Richard Madden, Nicola Fortune and Julie Gordon
Health Statistics in Australia: What We Know and Do Not Know
Reprinted from: *Int. J. Environ. Res. Public Health* **2022**, *19*, 4959, doi:10.3390/ijerph19094959 . . . 1

Ian Ring and Kalinda Griffiths
Australian Aboriginal and Torres Strait Islander Health Information: Progress, Pitfalls, and Prospects
Reprinted from: *Int. J. Environ. Res. Public Health* **2021**, *18*, 10274, doi:10.3390/ijerph181910274 . 13

James Eynstone-Hinkins and Lauren Moran
Enhancing Australian Mortality Data to Meet Future Health Information Demands
Reprinted from: *Int. J. Environ. Res. Public Health* **2022**, *19*, 603, doi:10.3390/ijerph19010603 . . . 29

Nicola Fortune, Rosamond H. Madden and Shane Clifton
Health and Access to Health Services for People with Disability in Australia: Data and Data Gaps
Reprinted from: *Int. J. Environ. Res. Public Health* **2021**, *18*, 11705, doi:10.3390/ijerph182111705 . 35

Julie Gordon, Helena Britt, Graeme C. Miller, Joan Henderson, Anthony Scott and Christopher Harrison
General Practice Statistics in Australia: Pushing a Round Peg into a Square Hole
Reprinted from: *Int. J. Environ. Res. Public Health* **2022**, *19*, 1912, doi:10.3390/ijerph19041912 . . . 51

Merran Smith and Felicity Flack
Data Linkage in Australia: The First 50 Years
Reprinted from: *Int. J. Environ. Res. Public Health* **2021**, *18*, 11339, doi:10.3390/ijerph182111339 . 61

Linda R. Jensen
Using Data Integration to Improve Health and Welfare Insights
Reprinted from: *Int. J. Environ. Res. Public Health* **2022**, *19*, 836, doi:10.3390/ijerph19020836 . . . 71

Sallie-Anne Pearson, Nicole Pratt, Juliana de Oliveira Costa, Helga Zoega, Tracey-Lea Laba, Christopher Etherton-Beer, Frank M. Sanfilippo, Alice Morgan, Lisa Kalisch Ellett, Claudia Bruno, Erin Kelty, Maarten IJzerman, David B. Preen, Claire M. Vajdic and David Henry
Generating Real-World Evidence on the Quality Use, Benefits and Safety of Medicines in Australia: History, Challenges and a Roadmap for the Future
Reprinted from: *Int. J. Environ. Res. Public Health* **2021**, *18*, 13345, doi:10.3390/ijerph182413345 . 81

Najith Amarasena, Sergio Chrisopoulos, Lisa M. Jamieson and Liana Luzzi
Oral Health of Australian Adults: Distribution and Time Trends of Dental Caries, Periodontal Disease and Tooth Loss
Reprinted from: *Int. J. Environ. Res. Public Health* **2021**, *18*, 11539, doi:10.3390/ijerph182111539 . 101

Sebastian Rosenberg, Luis Salvador-Carulla, Graham Meadows and Ian Hickie
Fit for Purpose—Re-Designing Australia's Mental Health Information System
Reprinted from: *Int. J. Environ. Res. Public Health* **2022**, *19*, 4808, doi:10.3390/ijerph19084808 . . . 115

Sonam Shelly, Emily Lodge, Carly Heyman, Felicity Summers, Amy Young, Jennifer Brew and Matthew James
Mental Health Services Data Dashboards for Reporting to Australian Governments during COVID-19
Reprinted from: *Int. J. Environ. Res. Public Health* **2021**, *18*, 10514, doi:10.3390/ijerph181910514 . **129**

John R. Goss
Health Expenditure Data, Analysis and Policy Relevance in Australia, 1967 to 2020
Reprinted from: *Int. J. Environ. Res. Public Health* **2022**, *19*, 2143, doi:10.3390/ijerph19042143 . . . **141**

Preface to "Health Statistics: The Australian Experience and Opportunities"

Health statistics have progressed dramatically in Australia since the 1980s when the Australian Government created the Australian Institute of Health. The 12 papers in this Special Issue describe these developments across a diverse range of topics, as well as providing an overview of the scope of health statistics in Australia and describing some ongoing gaps and problems.

It is hoped the papers will be of interest to international readers seeking to improve statistics about their health systems. Each country has its own approach to health and health service delivery and financing. In developing health statistics, the need to respect individuals' personal information, and for data standards, adequate resourcing and committed staffing are issues all countries face; the Australian experience provides valuable insights and examples. Australians will benefit from a comprehensive account of what has been achieved and what remains to be addressed. The papers in the Special Issue demonstrate the importance of continuing commitment to the statistical effort.

Thanks are due to all the authors for taking time from other pressing commitments to write these papers. Authors were chosen because of their known expertise in their respective fields, and it has been a pleasure and a privilege to cooperate with them. Nicola Fortune and Julie Gordon provided great help and skill in working with the authors, as well as contributing as authors themselves. Imelda Noti worked tirelessly so that deadlines were met, and the inevitable problems were efficiently resolved. Finally, thanks to the Journal's staff for their encouragement and tolerance throughout.

Richard Madden
Editor

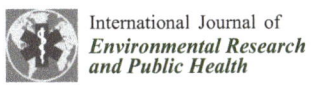

Review

Health Statistics in Australia: What We Know and Do Not Know

Richard Madden [1,*], Nicola Fortune [2,3] and Julie Gordon [4]

1. Faculty of Medicine and Health, University of Sydney, Sydney, NSW 2006, Australia
2. Centre for Disability Research and Policy, University of Sydney, Sydney, NSW 2006, Australia; nicola.fortune@sydney.edu.au
3. Centre of Research Excellence in Disability and Health, University of Melbourne, Carlton, VIC 3053, Australia
4. WHO Collaborating Centre for Strengthening Rehabilitation Capacity in Health Systems, University of Sydney, Sydney, NSW 2006, Australia; julie.gordon@sydney.edu.au
* Correspondence: richard.madden@sydney.edu.au

Abstract: Australia is a federation of six states and two territories (the States). These eight governmental entities share responsibility for health and health services with the Australian Government. Mortality statistics, including causes of death, have been collected since the late 19th century, with national data produced by the (now) Australian Bureau of Statistics (ABS) from 1907. Each State introduced hospital in-patient statistics, assisted by State offices of the ABS. Beginning in the 1970s, the ABS conducts regular health surveys, including specific collections on Aboriginal and Torres Strait Islander peoples. Overall, Australia now has a comprehensive array of health statistics, published regularly without political or commercial interference. Privacy and confidentiality are guaranteed by legislation. Data linkage has grown and become widespread. However, there are gaps, as papers in this issue demonstrate. Most notably, data on primary care patients and encounters reveal stark gaps. This paper accompanies a range of papers from expert authors across the health statistics spectrum in Australia. It is hoped that the collection of papers will inform interested readers and stand as a comprehensive review of the strengths and weaknesses of Australian health statistics in the early 2020s.

Keywords: health statistics; Australian health system; health surveys; Indigenous; data linkage

Citation: Madden, R.; Fortune, N.; Gordon, J. Health Statistics in Australia: What We Know and Do Not Know. *Int. J. Environ. Res. Public Health* **2022**, *19*, 4959. https://doi.org/10.3390/ijerph19094959

Academic Editors: Gabriel Gulis and Paul B. Tchounwou

Received: 14 December 2021
Accepted: 2 February 2022
Published: 19 April 2022

Publisher's Note: MDPI stays neutral with regard to jurisdictional claims in published maps and institutional affiliations.

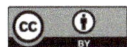

Copyright: © 2022 by the authors. Licensee MDPI, Basel, Switzerland. This article is an open access article distributed under the terms and conditions of the Creative Commons Attribution (CC BY) license (https://creativecommons.org/licenses/by/4.0/).

1. Introduction

Australia is a federation of six states and two self-governing territories (the Australian Capital Territory and the Northern Territory), referred to in this paper for simplicity as 'the States'. These eight governmental entities share responsibility for health and health services with the Australian (Commonwealth) Government. Many health services are provided by governments, with the private sector also delivering services, notably in primary care, dentistry, private hospitals, and pharmacy. Health constitutes some 10% of the Australian economy [1] (p. 173).

Australia introduced a system of universal health insurance (now known as Medicare) in the 1970s and 1980s. This covered privately provided medical services and shared the funding of public hospitals between the Australian and State governments [2]. As a result, there was a need to know much more about the services that the Australian health system delivered across its many arms. The decades that followed have seen great progress in building a national health information infrastructure to inform health policy, resource allocation, and delivery of health care across the nation. That work continues.

This paper is a commentary that aims to briefly describe the main components of Australia's health statistics system, highlight its breadth, successes, and novel features, point out some limitations, and indicate directions for future development. It provides a succinct overview of the current state of health statistics in Australia, set within a historical context, to inform future work to improve and build on Australia's health information infrastructure, and to demonstrate the crucial role of health statistics in running an effective and responsive health system.

In preparing this commentary, we have drawn upon a broad range of reports, technical documents, and other resources available on the websites of Australia's two main national statistics agencies (the Australian Bureau of Statistics and the Australian Institute of Health and Welfare) and the Australian Department of Health. The paper accompanies, and is informed by, a range of papers from expert authors across the health statistics spectrum in Australia. It is hoped that the collection of papers will inform interested readers and stand as a comprehensive review of the strengths and weaknesses of Australian health statistics in the early 2020s.

2. Australia's Statistical Agencies

Health statistics in Australia come, in large part, from two official statistics agencies—the Australian Bureau of Statistics and the Australian Institute of Health and Welfare. Both agencies are apolitical and explicitly serve all sectors of the community. Their values accord with the UN Fundamental Principles of Official Statistics [3], which state, as Principle 1, 'Official statistics provide an indispensable element in the information system of a democratic society, serving the Government, the economy and the public with data about the economic, demographic, social and environmental situation'. Principle 1 goes on to emphasise the need for impartiality and that statistics should be of 'practical utility'.

The (now) Australian Bureau of Statistics (ABS) dates from 1905, as the national statistics agency. It conducts a population census every five years, processes and publishes vital statistics, and conducts a range of social surveys, including in health. In 1987, the (now) Australian Institute of Health and Welfare (AIHW) was established to focus on health and community services statistics, especially using administrative data provided by the States. The AIHW works in conjunction with the ABS. Both agencies operate under national legislation which strictly protects the confidentiality and privacy of individual data [4,5]. The AIHW is required to report to Parliament on the state of Australia's health and health services every two years, in a publication called *Australia's Health*, beginning in 1988, with the most recent in 2020 [1].

3. Development of Health Statistics

This paper gives a brief description of various categories of health statistics in Australia, beginning with an outline of developments from the beginning of the 20th century. Sources of health statistics include patient and administrative data, surveys, and clinical registries.

Mortality statistics, including causes of death, have been collected since the late 19th century, with national data produced by the ABS from 1907.

Each State established a hospital in-patient data collection by the 1970s. Data on each patient episode was provided by the hospital to the State central collection. On its establishment, the first task for the AIHW was to produce national hospital in-patient statistics. This was a vital need as, under Medicare, funding of hospitals was now shared by the Commonwealth and States.

To pursue its charter, to bring together State health data into national collections, the AIHW led the development of the National Health Information Agreement in 1992. Under this agreement, all States agreed to establish national minimum datasets for key services, including hospital in-patients, and provide annual data to the AIHW for collation and publication. National minimum dataset specifications were developed, data standards were published in the National Health Data Dictionary (available in electronic form from July 1997) and, in the early 2000s, AIHW established a national online metadata registry for health, housing, and community services statistics and information (METeOR) [6].

National Health Information Plans were developed in 1995 and 2002 [7,8], to identify agreed priorities for national developments in health statistics. Development of a new National Health Information Strategy began in 2019 [9] but was not completed before national health governance arrangements changed in the light of the COVID-19 pandemic. This paper refers to the priorities of the 2002 plan, many of which remain just as relevant today.

Australia follows international standards for data collection and analysis where these exist, notably for causes of death (World Health Organization (WHO)) [10] and health expenditure (Organisation for Economic Co-operation and Development (OECD)) [11]. The AIHW is the Australian Collaborating Centre for the WHO's Family of International Classifications, the focus for Australian work on the development and maintenance of health classifications.

Australia's health statistics are financed through a variety of arrangements, including national direct funding of AIHW and ABS, contract funding by Australian Government departments, and State health department funding for administrative data and some special-purpose collections.

4. Health Surveys

The ABS conducted its first National Health Survey in 1977–1978, and these surveys have been repeated at regular intervals. In 2011, a National Nutrition and Physical Activity Survey and a National Health Measures Survey were added, providing biomedical information, in addition to self-reported information on health conditions such as cardiovascular disease, diabetes, kidney function, and risk factors.

The first of now regular National Aboriginal and Torres Strait Islander Health Surveys was conducted in 2004 [12]. Some health data are also collected in National Aboriginal and Torres Strait Islander Social Surveys [13].

In addition to these national health surveys, the AIHW has conducted a regular National Drug Strategy Household Survey, beginning in 1985, gathering information on the use of alcohol, tobacco, and illicit drugs [14].

The ABS conducted a National Survey of Mental Health and Wellbeing in 2007, giving a one-off view of the characteristics of people with mental health conditions (employment, housing, etc.) [15].

In 2019–2020, the ABS conducted a Patient Experiences Survey, covering health service use and experiences with health providers, as part of its annual Multipurpose Household Survey [16].

5. Health Statistics for Aboriginal and Torres Strait Islander Peopless

Australia has generally high health status, but notably, Aboriginal and Torres Strait Islander (Indigenous) people experience disadvantages, compared with other Australians, across a range of health outcomes [17].

Up to 1988, statistics on the health of Australia's Aboriginal and Torres Strait Islander people were almost non-existent. Australia became a nation in 1901. Its Constitution specified that 'Aboriginal natives' were not to be included in population estimates. This now-shocking provision ensured that there was little effort on statistics for the Indigenous population. Population estimates were conducted administratively, almost certainly underestimating the actual Indigenous population [18]. The exclusion provision was removed from the Constitution in 1967, and data about Indigenous status have been available since the 1971 Census, with Indigenous identification steadily improving over time [18].

In 1988, the first edition of AIHW's biennial report, *Australia's Health*, brought together an array of data to demonstrate the poor health status of Indigenous Australians.

The release of the first National Aboriginal and Torres Strait Islander Survey by the ABS in 1994 [19] marked a considerable step forward by producing a wide range of information on Indigenous people. The survey captured data on positive aspects of Indigenous life and culture, such as connection to land, as well as highlighting the systemic and intergenerational problems Indigenous people live with, including historical separation of children from families.

From 1996 on, the AIHW and ABS have worked in collaboration with Indigenous people to improve information on Indigenous health. A highlight was the release in 1997 of the first edition of *The Health and Welfare of Australia's Aboriginal and Torres Strait Islander Peoples*, published jointly by the two agencies and launched by the Australian Governor-General [20].

The development of Indigenous health statistics was the number one priority of the 2002 National Health Information Plan [8].

The development of Indigenous health statistics in Australia and many challenging issues are described by Ring and Griffiths [21] in this issue. The continuing, nationally acknowledged but persistent 'gap' between the health of Indigenous people and that of other Australians is highlighted each year in national 'Closing the Gap' reports [22]. Indigenous health statistics will remain a priority for development and a focus for lively debate into the future. Indigenous people are increasingly leading the development of new Indigenous controlled data and pushing the national statistical agencies to redouble their efforts.

6. Mortality

Each Australian state requires registration of deaths that occur in that state, using a standard death certificate that is aligned with international requirements set by the World Health Organization. Data on causes of death have been recorded in line with the International Classification of Diseases (ICD) since 1907, with over 100 years of causes of death available for analysis.

In 2006, the AIHW published *Mortality over the twentieth century in Australia* [23]. This publication showed the path of key diseases over the 20th century. For example, the female death rate for cancer did not vary much over the century, at 150 deaths per 100,000 population, although the composition changed, with lung cancer rising sharply, while cancers of the stomach, cervix, and uterus fell. The male cancer death rate increased from 166 deaths per 100,000 population in 1907 to 287 in 1985 and then fell to 247 by the year 2000, with lung cancer being the major varying cause of death. The male death rate for circulatory diseases increased from 437 deaths per 100,000 population in 1907 to 1020 in 1968, before falling to 319 in 2000.

Cause-of-death coding for Australia is centralised at the ABS in Brisbane (using internationally developed automated software), facilitating the development of specialist skills. For the past 15 years, the ABS has worked closely with State registrars and the National Coronial Information System (NCIS), which collates causes of death for all deaths referred to coroners across Australia and New Zealand. One particular result of this collaboration is much more complete data on deaths by suicide. The ABS now revises causes of death where updated information becomes available from coronial investigations which can take several years, and deaths can be coded as suicides based on the information in the NCIS.

The paper by Eynstone-Hinkins and Moran [24] in this issue provides up-to-date information on Australian mortality statistics, including COVID-19 deaths.

7. Hospital Treatment

As already described, a national collection of hospital in-patient data was the first task of the AIHW on its establishment in 1987. A national minimum dataset was introduced in 1990. Annual data have been published since 1993–1994, and the reporting has become progressively more timely. The collection covers patients in public and private hospitals [25].

Statistics on emergency department presentations are also produced, including principal diagnosis and triage category, as well as demographic characteristics of patients.

Non-inpatient data remain limited to administrative characteristics, with no information yet available on reasons for encounter, diagnoses, or interventions.

Hospital in-patient data have formed the information base for many important health policy developments at national and state levels, including in relation to casemix funding for hospitals, potentially preventable hospitalisation, and quality and safety developments in hospitals. Additionally, equity issues around hospital access and variations in intervention patterns can be explored.

7.1. Casemix Funding

Casemix funding was developed at a national level from the 1980s and was first introduced in Victoria in 1993. Casemix is now referred to in Australia as activity-based funding. Australia adopted the casemix models originally developed in the United States [26]. Casemix is a measure of hospital output for each patient, based on their diagnoses and interventions provided.

The Australian casemix system for acute in-patients (Australian Refined Diagnosis Related Groups) is based on hospital in-patient statistics and a hospital costing survey. The classifications used are an Australian modification of ICD-10 for diagnoses (ICD-10-AM) and the Australian Classification of Health Interventions (ACHI). Supplementary systems exist for sub-acute patients such as rehabilitation and palliative care.

The Australian activity-based funding system, including its supporting classifications, is not in the public domain. Several countries have licences from the Australian Government to use the system in their countries.

7.2. Potentially Preventable Hospitalisation

Potentially preventable hospitalisation is an indicator of the effectiveness of primary care. There is a range of vaccine-preventable, acute, and chronic conditions for which policymakers believe hospitalisation could be prevented by earlier community-based care, particularly significant diagnoses of interest include complications of diabetes and chronic obstructive pulmonary syndrome (COPD) [1] (Section 5). This is an example where statistics from one sector of the health system can be used as a performance indicator for another sector.

7.3. Quality and Safety

Selected diagnoses relating to 'hospital-acquired complications' are used as indicators of quality and safety issues in Australian hospitals [27]. There are 16 complications, including pressure injuries, health-care-associated infections, and respiratory complications. Hospital funding arrangements now include an adjustment for hospital-acquired complications, taking into account the non-preventable occurrences of these conditions.

Regrettably, there is duplication of hospital in-patient data collections. The Independent Hospitals Pricing Authority collects data from the States for its activity-based funding (casemix) functions. The Australian Department of Health collects clinical, demographic, and financial information for privately insured in-patients from private health insurers, and, through the Australian Private Hospital Data Bureau, also collects data from private hospitals covering patient demographics, clinical information, and hospital charges. The AIHW's collection covers most of the data items collected in these collections, apart from information on charges to private patients.

8. Primary Health Care

In contrast to information on hospital in-patients, primary health care statistics have had a chequered history and are a significant weak point in Australian health statistics. Primary health care practitioners, including general practitioners (GPs), nurses, allied health professionals, pharmacists, dentists, and Aboriginal and Torres Strait Islander health workers, provide services in a range of community settings and are critical first points of contact with the health system.

In 1998, a national sample-based data collection of general practice encounters (BEACH) was put in place by the University of Sydney and the AIHW, with wide-ranging support from general practitioners' professional representative groups and in partnership with a number of pharmaceutical companies. This unique partnership offered a publicly accessible dataset and provided information to participating pharmaceutical companies on their products' uses. The paper by Gordon et al. [28] in this issue outlines the development and uses of this data collection.

The Australian Government terminated funding for the BEACH collection in 2016 at short notice and without an alternative data collection in place. Currently, general practice statistical data are limited to extracts from GPs' electronic records, which come from multiple systems without any common data architecture or standards [29]. The samples drawn are not always structured to enable the production of statistics about all elements of the population, especially those with significant health disadvantages, such as Indigenous Australians. The AIHW is leading the development of a National Primary Health Care Data Asset [30] of which statistics about general practice are one component.

9. Public Health

In 1999, a National Public Health Information Plan was published, which focused on the need for improving national health surveys. As a result, information on a range of risk factors has been expanded and systematised over the past 20 years—smoking, alcohol use, exercise, and diet are examples.

The *Australia's Health* series reports on a range of population health indicators, as well as information on national screening programs. Between 2010 and 2013, Australia had a specialist agency focusing on preventive health. It produced a national report, *State of Preventive Health 2013* [31], which has not been repeated. This report brought together the national data on major risk factors, as well as international comparisons.

The National Notifiable Diseases Surveillance System brings together reports on notifiable diseases across Australia. Fortnightly reports are produced. Notifications in respect of Indigenous people made up more than half of the 330,000 notifications in 2016, the latest report available [32].

COVID-19 has seen separate and timely reporting of data on infection cases, hospitalisations, and deaths. It remains to be seen whether this results in the quality and timeliness of notifiable diseases information being improved and strengthened.

10. Mental Health

The paper in this issue by Rosenberg et al. [33] describes the development of mental health statistics since the 1990s. This development occurred outside the processes established under the National Health Information Agreement, even though the Australian Government and State health agencies were cooperating through their mental health experts. A separate governance arrangement was established through the Mental Health Information Strategy Sub-Committee.

The AIHW publishes an annual review of mental health services and associated resources in Australia [34,35]. Data are drawn from across AIHW data collections and other sources, including the 2007 ABS National Survey of Mental Health and Wellbeing.

11. Medicines: Use and Outcomes

Comprehensive data on medicines provided to Australians in the community are available from the national Pharmaceutical Benefits Scheme (PBS), established in 1948. Medicines below the cost threshold for the PBS and those provided to public hospital in-patients are not included in the PBS.

The use of these data for pharmaco-epidemiological purposes is described by Pearson et al. [36] in this issue. Increasingly, medicines data are linked to other national datasets (see Section 15, Data Linkage, below). The authors note that studies in Australia are relatively few and do not utilise all of the datasets available; they explore possible paths to facilitate a leap forward in medicine outcome studies.

12. Data on Health and Health Disadvantage for Particular Population Groups

There have been several references already in this paper to health statistics concerning Indigenous Australians. There are other population groups whose health status and access to health services also need to be monitored, as they experience significant disadvantages in relation to health.

People with disability are one such group. Statistics on people with disability and disability support services have been greatly improved over the past 20 years, although the introduction of the National Disability Insurance Scheme, itself a major social reform, has led to a break in the series of nationally consistent data on disability services, which was collected through the Disability Services National Minimum Dataset from 1991 to 2019 [37]. However, information on the health of people with disability and their access to health services has generally come from health and disability surveys, rather than from health services statistics. The paper by Fortune et al. [38] in this issue discusses this in more detail.

Medicare, Australia's universal health insurance system, gives all Australians the capacity to access high-quality medical and hospital services. The reality is that there is a clear excess burden of disease for lower socio-economic groups, notably in coronary heart disease, lung cancer, chronic kidney disease, and COPD [39]. In addition to survey evidence, data linkage is facilitating the examination of socio-economic variables in relation to health. For example, the ABS now links mortality data and census records, which has allowed examination of mortality due to various health conditions according to household equivalised income, highest educational attainment, and housing tenure [40].

Australia has about a quarter of its population born overseas, and almost half have at least one parent born overseas [41] (p. 271). Many health data collections include country of birth and language spoken at home. However, the AIHW has acknowledged that information on culturally and linguistically diverse (CALD) populations is among Australia's data gaps [1] (p. 6). *Australia's Health 2020* omitted data on CALD populations altogether. The 2018 edition briefly discussed the generally lower age-standardised mortality rates and rates of potentially preventable hospitalisations for people born outside Australia, compared with the Australian-born population. These data gaps have been thoroughly addressed in a recent report by the Federation of Ethnic Communities Councils of Australia (FECCA) [42].

In Australia, prisons and corrective services are the responsibility of the States. Without Australian Government involvement, it took many years for a national effort to report on the health of prisoners, which is the responsibility of State health departments or State correctional services agencies. Since 2009, the AIHW has conducted the National Prisoner Health Data Collection every 3 years. Data reported highlight significant mental health problems, high rates of smoking and drug use, and a high prevalence of disability among prisoners [43].

13. Health Registries

Each Australian State has operated a cancer registry for many years. The AIHW maintains the National Cancer Statistics Clearing House (NCSCH), which was established in 1986 as the national repository of cancer incidence and mortality statistics. The repository is used to produce national cancer statistics. Each jurisdiction uses the national minimum dataset for its reporting. In addition, the jurisdictions collaborate with the AIHW to produce registries for breast, cervical, and bowel cancer screening.

There is now a wide range of clinical registries in Australia. These include clinical quality, disease, immunisation, and product registries. A Framework for clinical quality registries has been developed by the Australian Commission on Safety and Quality in Health Care [44].

14. Oral Health

Dental statistics have been well developed in Australia through a specialist centre at the University of Adelaide, which has worked in collaboration with AIHW. Foundation work in South Australia was built to give a rich picture of child and adult dental health, as well as the dental health of Aboriginal and Torres Strait Islander peoples. The paper in this issue by Amarasena et al. [45] describes a recent national oral health survey and the changes in dental health over the past 30 years.

15. Data Linkage

Data linkage has been mentioned earlier in this paper. Data linkage involves the development of enriched datasets by linking two or more datasets. Data linkage in Australia commenced in Western Australia in the 1990s and now occurs in all State jurisdictions, and is supported by the Public Health Research Network (see Smith et al. in this issue) [46]. Ethical approval is essential for data linkage because linked data can readily produce identifiable data even if the original datasets are de-identified.

The AIHW, as described by Jensen [47] has developed the National Integrated Health Services Information Analysis Asset (NIHSIAA) linking a range of its datasets and other Australian Government datasets, thus bringing together data covering hospitals, Medicare, Pharmaceutical Benefits Scheme, Repatriation Pharmaceutical Benefits Scheme, residential aged care, and the National Death Index.

16. Financing

Australia has produced estimates of national health expenditure since 1980, following the OECD's guidelines. The paper by Goss [48] in this issue discusses this work and presents a fascinating dissection of the growth in Australia's health expenditure this century.

17. Workforce

From its commencement in 1987, the AIHW collated health workforce data from state registration authorities, with a focus on the medical and nursing workforce. At registration (then administered at the state level), individual practitioners were asked to provide demographic and employment information about themselves. The resulting statistics formed a valuable basis for workforce planning, highlighting urban/rural disparities in the medical workforce and the ageing of the nursing workforce.

In 2010, national health workforce registration was introduced through the National Registration and Accreditation Scheme, and responsibility for statistical reports remained with AIHW. In 2016, responsibility for workforce statistics was passed to the Australian Department of Health [44].

The AIHW produced comprehensive reports on the health and community services workforces after the 1996, 2001, and 2006 population censuses [49].

18. Discussion

The Australian health system encompasses a mix of Australian Government and State Government responsibilities and is a combination of public and private services. This complexity makes a national health statistics system essential if the Australian health sector is to be understood, accountable, responsive, and improved. Since the 1980s, this system has been established, developed, and maintained. All jurisdictions and sectors have contributed to this effort. The 1992 National Health Information Agreement (NHIA) provided a critical framework for the development of national datasets, ensuring common data standards have been adopted in these datasets. The contrast with health sectors that have stayed outside the NHIA arrangements is stark.

Australia now has a comprehensive array of health statistics, published regularly without political or commercial interference. Privacy and confidentiality are guaranteed by legislation.

However, there are gaps, as some papers in this issue illustrate; most notable are data on primary care patients and encounters, with no current reliable information on the reason for encounter, consultation outcome, and other aspects of primary health care. Similar gaps exist for patients treated by medical specialists outside hospitals, and for patients of allied health practitioners. Additionally, some datasets (such as health workforce) exist in silos, separate from the national statistical agencies where users would expect to find information readily accessible.

The utility of national health statistical collections is dependent on the development and widespread use of national minimum datasets, which ensure the supply of comparable data from different sectors (such as public and private hospitals) and jurisdictions. The more recent emergence of 'big data' sets and analysis provides new opportunities, as long as good statistical practices are followed [50] and high ethical and privacy standards are adhered to.

The papers in this issue highlight that health statistics must respond to health policy needs and developments, and to emerging health issues. Casemix funding for hospitals energised the development and supply of hospital statistics and now relies on them. COVID-19 has led to more timely incidence and mortality statistics and focused attention on the calculation of excess mortality in a pandemic [35].

Work on the postponed National Health Information Strategy should be resumed so that clear priorities for health statistics developments are identified and committed to by all stakeholders. National consultation had occurred prior to the deferral of the development in 2020, which naturally gave rise to wide-ranging demands for improved data and analysis. It is important that the strategy focuses on a few key areas with clear short- and medium-term priorities. These include the following aspects:

- Primary health care: Broad-ranging work on a National Primary Health Care Data Asset has been underway for some years by the AIHW. This appears to have an ambitious scope and needs to be seen as a project of long-term development. Immediate steps are needed to fill the gap left by the termination of the BEACH collection, with a robust, statistically reliable, and nationally representative collection. The limitations of generating statistics based on data extraction from GP electronic records must be acknowledged and addressed, as well as methods developed to overcome these.
- Disability: The development of a National Disability Data Asset is advancing, and significant funding was allocated by the Australian Government in late 2021. This development is broadly focused and relies mainly on the identification of people with disability through disability-specific services and payments. The ability to identify people with disability consistently within health service data systems is necessary for monitoring equity of access and outcomes. Creating a succinct question or short set of questions that can function as a disability 'identifier' for use in administrative data collections is a key priority.
- Mental health: Developments in this sector have occurred outside the mainstream structures under the National Health Information Agreement, so statistics in this crucial health sector remain separate from other health statistics. Data linkage provides a strong platform today to bring together data on services provided in the various sectors: primary health care, community care, and hospitals. The National Health Information Strategy development needs to prioritise mental health statistics and integrate them with other health statistics streams.
- Hospital in-patient statistics: The duplication of collections described above should be removed, with the national collection for public and private hospitals managed by the AIHW, which should prepare a common dataset for all other national agencies. While some additional data items would need to be added to the AIHW collection, one collection would replace four.

19. Conclusions

Australia has a robust and reliable set of health statistics. This is the result of many decades of national governance cooperation, resourcing, and effort. The ongoing commitment of resources and collaboration among stakeholders continues to be essential to ensure a robust evidence base to inform policy and practice, based on nationally consistent data standards, and to underpin research efforts, into the future. Some specific potential improvements have been highlighted, and the full potential of data linkage has yet to be achieved.

People provide information about themselves and their health in many settings and are often unaware that this information provides input to health statistics which, in turn, improves health and health services [47]. Respecting individuals' data remains at the heart of the health statistics effort, and using it as well as possible is a key responsibility for the statistical community.

Author Contributions: Conceptualization, R.M., N.F. and J.G.; investigation, R.M., N.F., J.G.; writing—review and editing, R.M., N.F., J.G. All authors have read and agreed to the published version of the manuscript.

Funding: This research received no external funding.

Institutional Review Board Statement: Not applicable.

Informed Consent Statement: Not applicable.

Data Availability Statement: Not applicable.

Conflicts of Interest: The authors declare no conflict of interest.

References

1. Australian Institute of Health and Welfare. *Australia's Health 2020 Data Insights*; Australia's Health Series no. 17 Cat. no: AUS 231; AIHW: Canberra, Australia, 2020.
2. Scotton, R.B.; MacDonald, C.R. *The Making of Medibank*; School of Health Services Management, University of New South Wales: Sydney, Australia, 1993; p. 320.
3. United Nations. Fundamental Principles of Official Statistics (A/RES/68/261 from 29 January 2014). Available online: https://unstats.un.org/fpos/ (accessed on 7 September 2021).
4. Australian Bureau of Statistics Act 1975. Available online: https://www.legislation.gov.au/Details/C2019C00184 (accessed on 15 September 2021).
5. Australian Institute of Health and Welfare Act 1987. Available online: www.legislation.gov.au/Details/C2018C00474 (accessed on 15 September 2021).
6. Australian Institute of Health and Welfare. METeOR Metadata Online Registry. Available online: https://meteor.aihw.gov.au/content/index.phtml/itemId/181162 (accessed on 15 September 2021).
7. AIHW and Australian Health Ministers' Advisory Council. *National Health Information Development Plan*; Australian Government: Canberra, Australia, 1995.
8. National Health Information Management Group. *Health Information Development Priorities*; AIHW: Canberra, Australia, 2003.
9. Australian Institute of Health and Welfare. *2019–2020 Annual Report*; AIHW: Canberra, Australia, 2020.
10. World Health Organization. *International Statistical Classification of Diseases and Related Health Problems*, 5th ed.; 10th Revision, Instruction Manual; WHO: Geneva, Switzerland, 2016.
11. OECD; Eurostat; World Health Organization. *A System of Health Accounts 2011*; Revised Edition; OECD Publishing: Paris, France, 2017. [CrossRef]
12. Australian Bureau of Statistics (2018–2019 Financial Year) National Aboriginal and Torres Strait Islander Health Survey. Available online: https://www.abs.gov.au/statistics/people/aboriginal-and-torres-strait-islander-peoples/national-aboriginal-and-torres-strait-islander-health-survey/latest-release (accessed on 25 September 2021).
13. Australian Bureau of Statistics (2016). 4714.0—National Aboriginal and Torres Strait Islander Social Survey, 2014–2015. Available online: https://www.abs.gov.au/AUSSTATS/abs@.nsf/Lookup/4714.0Main+Features100022014-15?OpenDocument (accessed on 25 September 2021).
14. Australian Institute of Health and Welfare. National Drug Strategy Household Survey 2019. Available online: https://www.aihw.gov.au/about-our-data/our-data-collections/national-drug-strategy-household-survey/2019-ndshs (accessed on 25 September 2021).

15. Australian Bureau of Statistics 2008. National Survey of Mental Health and Wellbeing: Summary of Results. Available online: https://www.abs.gov.au/statistics/health/mental-health/national-survey-mental-health-and-wellbeing-summary-results/latest-release (accessed on 29 November 2021).
16. Australian Bureau of Statistics (2019-20 Financial Year). Patient Experiences in Australia: Summary of Findings. Available online: https://www.abs.gov.au/statistics/health/health-services/patient-experiences-australia-summary-findings/latest-release (accessed on 25 September 2021).
17. Australian Institute of Health and Welfare. Indigenous Health and Wellbeing, Australia's Health 2020. Available online: https://www.aihw.gov.au/reports/australias-health/indigenous-health-and-wellbeing (accessed on 20 September 2021).
18. Madden, R.C.; Pulver, L.R.J. Aboriginal and Torres Strait Islander Population: More Than Reported. *Aust. Actuar. J. (AAJ)* **2009**, *15*, 181–208.
19. Australian Bureau of Statistics. *1994 National Aboriginal and Torres Strait Islander Survey (NATSIS)*; ABS: Canberra, Australia, 1994.
20. Australian Bureau of Statistics; Australian Institute of Health and Welfare. *The Health and Welfare of Australia's Aboriginal and Torres Strait Islander Peoples*; Commonwealth of Australia: Canberra, Australia, 1997.
21. Ring, I.; Griffiths, K. Australian Aboriginal and Torres Strait Islander Health Information: Progress, Pitfalls, and Prospects. *Int. J. Environ. Res. Public Health* **2021**, *18*, 10274. [CrossRef] [PubMed]
22. Productivity Commission. *Closing the Gap Annual Data Compilation Report*; Commonwealth of Australia: Canberra, Australia, 2021.
23. Australian Institute of Health and Welfare. Mortality over the twentieth century in Australia. In *Trends and Patterns in Major Causes of Death. Mortality Surveillance Series no 4*; AIHW cat. no. PHE 73; AIHW: Canberra, Australia, 2006.
24. Eynstone-Hinkins, J.; Moran, L. Enhancing Australian Mortality Data to Meet Future Health Information Demands. *Int. J. Environ. Res. Public Health* **2022**, *19*, 603. [CrossRef] [PubMed]
25. Australian Institute of Health and Welfare. National Hospitals Data Collection. Available online: https://www.aihw.gov.au/about-our-data/our-data-collections/national-hospitals-data-collection (accessed on 20 September 2021).
26. Duckett, S.J. Hospital payment arrangements to encourage efficiency: The case of Victoria, Australia. *Health Policy (Amsterdam)* **1995**, *34*, 113–134. [CrossRef]
27. Australian Commission on Safety and Quality in Health Care. Hospital Acquired Complications. Available online: https://www.safetyandquality.gov.au/our-work/indicators/hospital-acquired-complications (accessed on 20 September 2021).
28. Gordon, J.; Britt, H.; Miller, G.C.; Henderson, J.; Scott, A.; Harrison, C. General Practice Statistics in Australia: Pushing a Round Peg into a Square Hole. *Int. J. Environ. Res. Public Health* **2022**, *19*, 1912. [CrossRef]
29. Busingye, D.; Gianacas, C.; Pollack, A.; Chidwick, K.; Merrifield, A.; Norman, S.; Mullin, B.; Hayhurst, R.; Blogg, S.; Havard, A.; et al. Data Resource Profile: MedicineInsight, an Australian national primary health care database. *Int. J. Epidemiol.* **2019**, *48*, 1741. [CrossRef] [PubMed]
30. Australian Institute of Health and Welfare. Primary Health Care Data Development. Available online: https://www.aihw.gov.au/reports-data/health-welfare-services/primary-health-care/primary-health-care-data-development (accessed on 29 November 2021).
31. Australian National Preventive Health Agency. *State of Preventative Health 2013. Report to the Australian Government Minister for Health*; Commonwealth of Australia: Canberra, Australia, 2013.
32. Communicable Diseases Intelligence. *Australia's Notifiable Disease Status, 2016: Annual Report of the National Notifiable Diseases Surveillance System. Communicable Diseases Intelligence, Vol 45. Commonwealth of Australia as Represented by the Department of Health*; Australian Department of Health: Canberra, Australia, 2021. [CrossRef]
33. Rosenberg, S.; Salvador-Carulla, L.; Meadows, G.; Hickie, I. Fit for Purpose—Re-Designing Australia's Mental Health Information System. *Int. J. Environ. Res. Public Health* **2022**, *19*, 4808. [CrossRef]
34. Australian Institute of Health and Welfare. Mental health services in Australia 2021. Available online: https://www.aihw.gov.au/reports/mental-health-services/mental-health-services-in-australia/report-contents/summary-of-mental-health-services-in-australia (accessed on 26 September 2021).
35. Shelly, S.; Lodge, E.; Heyman, C.; Summers, F.; Young, A.; Brew, J.; James, M. Mental Health Services Data Dashboards for Reporting to Australian Governments during COVID-19. *Int. J. Environ. Res. Public Health* **2021**, *18*, 10514. [CrossRef] [PubMed]
36. Pearson, S.-A.; Pratt, N.; de Oliveira Costa, J.; Zoega, H.; Laba, T.-L.; Etherton-Beer, C.; Sanfilippo, F.M.; Morgan, A.; Kalisch Ellett, L.; Bruno, C.; et al. Generating Real-World Evidence on the Quality Use, Benefits and Safety of Medicines in Australia: History, Challenges and a Roadmap for the Future. *Int. J. Environ. Res. Public Health* **2021**, *18*, 13345. [CrossRef] [PubMed]
37. Australian Institute of Health and Welfare. *Disability Support Services: Services Provided under the National Disability Agreement 2018–19*; Bulletin no. 149. Cat. no. DIS 75; AIHW: Canberra, Australia, 2020.
38. Fortune, N.; Madden, R.H.; Clifton, S. Health and Access to Health Services for People with Disability in Australia: Data and Data Gaps. *Int. J. Environ. Res. Public Health* **2021**, *18*, 11705. [CrossRef] [PubMed]
39. Australian Institute of Health and Welfare. *Indicators of Socioeconomic Inequalities in Cardiovascular Disease, Diabetes and Chronic Kidney Disease*; Cat. no. CDK 12; AIHW: Canberra, Australia, 2019.
40. Tam, S.-M.; Clarke, F. Big Data, Official Statistics and Some Initiatives by the Australian Bureau of Statistics. *Int. Stat. Rev.* **2015**, *83*, 436–448. [CrossRef]
41. Australian Institute of Health and Welfare. *Australia's Health 2018*; Australia's Health Series no. 16 AUS 221; AIHW: Canberra, Australia, 2018.

42. Federation of Ethnic Communities Councils of Australia. If We Don't Count It... It Doesn't Count! Towards Consistent National Data Collection and Reporting on Cultural, Ethnic and Linguistic Diversity. Available online: https://fecca.org.au/if-we-dont-count-it-it-doesnt-count/ (accessed on 22 September 2021).
43. Australian Institute of Health and Welfare. *The Health of Australia's Prisoners*; Cat. no. PHE 246; AIHW: Canberra, Australia, 2019.
44. Department of Health, Australian Government. Doctors in Focus 2018. Available online: https://hwd.health.gov.au/resources/publications/factsheet-mdcl-2018-full.pdf (accessed on 20 September 2021).
45. Amarasena, N.; Chrisopoulos, S.; Jamieson, L.M.; Luzzi, L. Oral Health of Australian Adults: Distribution and Time Trends of Dental Caries, Periodontal Disease and Tooth Loss. *Int. J. Environ. Res. Public Health* **2021**, *18*, 11539. [CrossRef] [PubMed]
46. Smith, M.; Flack, F. Data Linkage in Australia: The First 50 Years. *Int. J. Environ. Res. Public Health* **2021**, *18*, 11339. [CrossRef] [PubMed]
47. Jensen, L.R. Using Data Integration to Improve Health and Welfare Insights. *Int. J. Environ. Res. Public Health* **2022**, *19*, 836. [CrossRef] [PubMed]
48. Goss, J.R. Health Expenditure Data, Analysis and Policy Relevance in Australia, 1967 to 2020. *Int. J. Environ. Res. Public Health* **2022**, *19*, 2143. [CrossRef] [PubMed]
49. Australian Institute of Health and Welfare. *Health and Community Services Labour Force 2006*; National Health Labour Force Series Number 42. Cat. no. HWL 43; AIHW: Canberra, Australia, 2009.
50. Daas, P.J.H.; Puts, M.J.; Buelens, B.; Hurk, P.A.M.v.d. Big Data as a Source for Official Statistics. *J. Off. Stat.* **2015**, *31*, 249–262. [CrossRef]

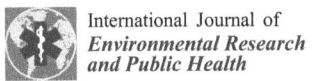

International Journal of *Environmental Research and Public Health*

Review

Australian Aboriginal and Torres Strait Islander Health Information: Progress, Pitfalls, and Prospects

Ian Ring [1,*] and Kalinda Griffiths [2]

1 Tropical Health and Medicine, James Cook University, Townsville 4810, Australia
2 Centre for Big Data Research in Health, Medicine, University of New South Wales, Sydney 2052, Australia; kalinda.griffiths@unsw.edu.au
* Correspondence: ian.ring@jcu.edu.au

Abstract: Despite significant developments in Aboriginal and Torres Strait Islander Health information over the last 25 years, many challenges remain. There are still uncertainties about the accuracy of estimates of the summary measure of life expectancy, and methods to estimate changes in life expectancy over time are unreliable because of changing patterns of identification. Far too little use is made of the wealth of information that is available, and formal systems for systematically using that information are often vestigial to non-existent. Available information has focussed largely on traditional biomedical topics and too little on access to, expenditure on, and availability of services required to improve health outcomes, and on the underpinning issues of social and emotional wellbeing. It is of concern that statistical artefacts may have been misrepresented as indicating real progress in key health indices. Challenges and opportunities for the future include improving the accuracy of estimation of life expectancy, provision of community level data, information on the availability and effectiveness of health services, measurement of the underpinning issues of racism, culture and social and emotional wellbeing (SEWB), enhancing the interoperability of data systems, and capacity building and mechanisms for Indigenous data governance. There is little point in having information unless it is used, and formal mechanisms for making full use of information in a proper policy/planning cycle are urgently required.

Keywords: Aboriginal and Torres Strait Islander health; Indigenous health measurement; life expectancy; misleading statistics; management use of information; data sovereignty; governance

Citation: Ring, I.; Griffiths, K. Australian Aboriginal and Torres Strait Islander Health Information: Progress, Pitfalls, and Prospects. *Int. J. Environ. Res. Public Health* **2021**, *18*, 10274. https://doi.org/10.3390/ijerph181910274

Academic Editor: Paul B. Tchounwou

Received: 24 August 2021
Accepted: 26 September 2021
Published: 29 September 2021

Publisher's Note: MDPI stays neutral with regard to jurisdictional claims in published maps and institutional affiliations.

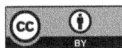

Copyright: © 2021 by the authors. Licensee MDPI, Basel, Switzerland. This article is an open access article distributed under the terms and conditions of the Creative Commons Attribution (CC BY) license (https://creativecommons.org/licenses/by/4.0/).

1. Progress

Thompson [1] and Smith [2] have described the early history of the development of Aboriginal and Torres Strait Islander health statistics. In brief, the National Health and Medical Research Council (NHMRC) in 1955 drew attention to the fact that despite reported high levels of Indigenous morbidity and mortality in parts of Australia, precise information was not available. The first regular collection of data was commenced by the Northern Territory (NT) administration on infant mortality in 1957, but that was the only systematic collection for many years. In 1973 Commonwealth and jurisdictional Health Ministers endorsed a policy of collecting national Aboriginal health statistics. Progress was painfully slow and in the early 1980s no jurisdiction identified Aboriginal and Torres Strait Islander people in birth and death records. This is despite the 1967 constitutional changes to include Aboriginal and Torres Strait Islander people in the national population count. In 1984 the Commonwealth established a high-level taskforce on Aboriginal health statistics, but progress with implementation of its recommendations to prioritise Indigenous identifiers in vital statistics and hospital and perinatal statistics by the jurisdictions was patchy. Responsibility then passed to the newly formed Australian Institute of Health (AIH), but the funds provided for progressing the development of Indigenous health statistics were only half of those recommended arising from the National Aboriginal Health Strategy (NAHS) in 1989.

There have been extensive developments in the capture of Aboriginal and Torres Strait Islander data for the purposes of national statistics in the last 60 years. Since federation, there have been a number of laws enacted for the purposes of identifying and counting Aboriginal and Torres Strait Islander people [3]. While there are departments, centres, and groups within the Australian government that focus on Aboriginal and Torres Strait Islander statistics, there have been some, but limited, developments in government support for Aboriginal and Torres Strait Islander oversight. Historically, it has often been individuals within government who have worked with Aboriginal and Torres Strait Islander communities and individuals to support the visibility of Indigenous people in the nation.

The Australian Bureau of Statistics (ABS) and the Australian Institute of Health and Welfare (AIHW) instituted a joint unit in Darwin in 1996. In 1997 this unit produced the first in a series of what was intended to be flagship biennial publications on the Health and Welfare of Australia's Aboriginal and Torres Strait Islander Peoples [4]. Importantly, the first edition was launched in Darwin by the Governor General of Australia, Sir William Deane, who emphasised the importance of good statistics to drive good policy and action:

"This report will hopefully do much to influence all Australians, both Indigenous and non-Indigenous, to approach the question of the health and welfare of Aboriginal and Torres Strait Islander peoples, particularly children, on the basis of unprejudiced statistical facts [5]."

The joint unit was disbanded after 7 years, and ABS and AIHW followed independent paths.

1.1. The Aboriginal and Torres Strait Islander Health Information Plan

It was in this context that the Aboriginal and Torres Strait Islander Health Information Plan was prepared for the Australian Health Ministers Advisory Council (AHMAC) by ABS and AIHW in 1997 [6], appropriately subtitled ... *This time let's make it happen*, and is a convenient starting point. The subtitle is an explicit recognition of the relative failure of previous attempts to make significant progress with this important topic. As the foreword to the report says:

In 1994 the AHMAC endorsed the recommendation of the national body responsible for national health information, that the highest national priority was to:

"Work with Aboriginal and Torres Strait Islander peoples to develop a plan to improve all aspects of information about their health and health services."

Funds were provided to implement that recommendation and develop a plan.

AHMAC accepted the recommendations of the Report and instructed the National Health Information Management Group (NHIMG) to oversee the implementation. NHIMG established an implementation group including Indigenous health organisations and other agencies for this purpose.

The report described the shortcomings in the collection, processing and use of Indigenous health information, and emphasized the central role of the poor quality of Indigenous identification in current collections. The report went on to say that there was little new in its findings and recommendations and noted the lack of commitment to implement the findings of the numerous reviews that had been undertaken as the chief reason for the overall lack of progress.

Up until the publication of this report, the main source of national information had been the National Aboriginal and Torres Strait Island Survey conducted by the ABS in 1994 [7]. This was as part of the Government's response to Recommendation 49 [8] of the Royal Commission into Aboriginal Deaths in Custody, "That proposals for a special national survey covering a range of social, demographic, health and economic circumstances of the Aboriginal population with full Aboriginal participation at all levels be supported". The aim was to provide Australian governments with a "stronger information base for planning for the empowerment of Australia's Indigenous peoples and for measuring progress in meeting their objectives, aspirations and needs".

1.2. National Advisory Group on Aboriginal and Torres Strait Islander Health Information and Data (NAGATSIHID)

NAGATSIHID was established "as a result of a decision by AHMAC in October 2000, to improve reporting on the health status of Indigenous Australians. It was set up as the national body to create a partnership between the Commonwealth, jurisdictions and Aboriginal and Torres Strait Islander people to improve Indigenous information in national and jurisdictional data collections" [9]. The purpose of the committee was to make strategic decisions regarding the use of government held data pertaining to Aboriginal and Torres Strait Islander people and work to improve the quality and accessibility of Indigenous data and information.

What made NAGATSIHID different from other committees was: "(i) the level of representation from the governments (chaired by an AHMAC member); (ii) it had a majority Aboriginal and Torres Strait Islander membership with representatives from a wide range of key stakeholders in Aboriginal and Torres Strait Islander health such as the community controlled sector, academia and the government sector with decision making made through an Aboriginal and Torres Strait Islander quorum; (iii) it provided a unique example of an effective working partnership between government agencies, Aboriginal and Torres Strait Islander people and organisations to advance the development and use of data and information on the health of Indigenous Australians; (iv) having a majority of Indigenous people on NAGATSIHID gave the agencies some confidence that the decisions by AHMAC (through NAGATSIHID) reflect the views of Indigenous people and their representative bodies; and (v) it is recognised internationally and has been responsible for many of the significant changes in Aboriginal and Torres Strait Islander health statistics and data" [9].

The main role of NAGATSIHID was "to provide broad strategic advice to AHMAC, and in particular was responsible for:

- Continuing the implementation of the 1997 Aboriginal and Torres Strait Islander health Information Plan—*this time let's make it happen* (AIHW 1997 [6]);
- Advising AIHW and ABS on information and data priorities;
- Providing advice to the Australian Government's Department of Health (DoH) on the Aboriginal and Torres Strait Islander Health Performance Framework (HPF)" [10].

NAGATSIHID was abolished in 2019, without notice to its members. While there are a number of advisory committees within government agencies [11,12] to support decision-making regarding Aboriginal and Torres Strait Islander data by those individual agencies, there has been no replacement to the principal committee.

1.3. Development of National Surveys

In 2001, the National Health Survey was enhanced with a supplementary sample of Indigenous people of sufficient size to produce national estimates for Indigenous people. The supplementary sample was part funded by the Commonwealth and the jurisdictions, and became the first national Indigenous health survey. This was followed by a larger supplementary Indigenous sample in 2004 to provide both national and jurisdictional estimates, and thereafter, was conducted every 6 years [13].

Even though a national biomedical risk factor survey had been conducted for the Australian administration in Papua New Guinea in the late 1960s [14], it was not until 2012–2013 that a parallel survey was conducted in Australia, and was made possible by additional funding provided by the Australian Government Department of Health and the National Heart Foundation of Australia. This national survey included two Indigenous components, a National Aboriginal and Torres Strait Islander Nutrition and Physical Activity Survey and a National Aboriginal and Torres Strait Islander Health Measures Survey [15].

1.4. ABS and AIHW Publications

Currently, the ABS has a range of publications concerning Aboriginal and Torres Strait Islander peoples, based largely on the census and the extensive ABS survey program [13] covering health surveys; population estimates and projections; life tables; understanding the increase in census counts; Torres Strait Islander people characteristics; Aboriginal and Torres Strait Islander women; smoking trends; education, etc.

The AIHW regularly produces a wide variety of publications on Indigenous health and welfare topics. Recent topics include: the Health Performance Framework; acute rheumatic fever and rheumatic heart disease; Indigenous injury deaths; Indigenous specific primary health care datasets: The Online Services Report and the national Key Performance Indicators; Northern Territory remote Aboriginal investment: oral health program; better cardiac care measures for Aboriginal and Torres Strait Islander people; cultural safety in health care for Indigenous Australians; hearing health outreach services for Aboriginal and Torres Strait Islander children in the Northern Territory; aged care; disability support; Indigenous community safety; Indigenous education and skills; Indigenous employment; Indigenous housing; Indigenous income and finance; understanding Indigenous welfare and wellbeing; Indigenous eye health; Indigenous mental health and suicide prevention clearinghouse, etc.

1.5. The Overcoming Indigenous Disadvantage (OID) Report

The Council of Australian Governments (COAG) commissioned the OID [16] report in 2002, and nominated two core objectives for the report:

- To inform Australian governments about whether policy programs and interventions are achieving improved outcomes for Aboriginal and Torres Strait Islander people;
- To be meaningful to Aboriginal and Torres Strait Islander people.

As the 2020 report [17] says, "This edition of the report seeks to identify the significant strengths of, and sources of wellbeing for, Aboriginal and Torres Strait Islander people—and to illustrate the nature of the disadvantage they experience, focusing on the key structural and systemic barriers that contribute to this disadvantage. The framework of indicators focuses on some of the factors that contributed to their wellbeing or that cause the disadvantage they experience, these factors were selected based on evidence, logic and where experience suggests that targeted policies will have the greatest impact. The indicators are supplemented by additional research on structural and systemic barriers that contribute to, or maintain, the disadvantage experienced by Aboriginal and Torres Strait Islander people, and where governments may have a role in removing barriers."

1.6. The Aboriginal and Torres Strait Islander Health Performance Framework

The purpose of this report is said to be that "The Aboriginal and Torres Strait Islander Health Performance Framework (HPF) monitors progress in Aboriginal and Torres Strait Islander health outcomes, health system performance and the broader determinants of health (such as employment, education and safety). The HPF is a comprehensive source of evidence designed to inform policy, planning, program development and research.

Beginning in 2006, HPF reports have been released every 2–3 years. The HPF includes data analysis drawn from over 60 data collections, findings from research and evaluations, and analysis of implications of the evidence for government, health services and the research sector.

The HPF consists of 68 measures across three domains (Tiers): Tier 1—Health status and outcomes; Tier 2—Determinants of health; Tier 3—Health system performance" [18].

1.7. Expenditure

The Indigenous Expenditure Report (IER) aims to contribute to better policy making and improved outcomes for Indigenous Australians and will

"3. include expenditure by both Commonwealth and State/Territory governments (and local government if possible), and over time will:

(a) Allow reporting on Indigenous and non-Indigenous social status and economic status;
(b) Include expenditure on Indigenous-specific and key mainstream programs;
(c) Be reconcilable with published government financial statistics.

4. focus on on-the-ground services in areas such as: education; justice; health; housing; community services; employment; and other significant expenditure

6. provide governments with a better understanding of the level and patterns of expenditure on services which support Indigenous Australians, and provide policy makers with an additional tool to target policies to Close the Gap in Indigenous Disadvantage" [19].

Reports have been produced periodically since 2010 with the most recent report being the 2017 version.

While the IER produced by the Productivity Commission focuses on government expenditure, expenditure analysis carried out by AIHW for the HPF "encompasses government, non-government, private and individual expenditure on health and medical services, hospital services (admitted and non-admitted patients), community health services, dental services, aids and appliances, pharmaceuticals, patient transport and public health programs . . . ". It points out that "four interacting factors within Australia's health system potentially have major consequences for the health of many Aboriginal and Torres Strait Islander people, namely limited Indigenous-specific primary health care services; Indigenous Australians' underutilisation of many mainstream health services and limited access to government health subsidies; increasing price signals in the public health system (such as co-payments) and a low Indigenous private health insurance rate; and failure to maintain real health expenditure levels over time" [20]. An important element of the AIHW expenditure analysis is that, unlike the IER, it includes non-government expenditure as well as government expenditure, allowing for a more meaningful comparison of Indigenous and non-Indigenous expenditure on health and social areas.

1.8. Indigenous Data Developments

A range of conversations and meetings to identify what is required for data to support the needs and aspirations of Aboriginal and Torres Strait Islander people have occurred more frequently over the past 5 years. Emerging from these discussions, Aboriginal and Torres Strait Islander people identified the need for strategic government and organisational partnerships to work towards the development of the data capabilities of Aboriginal and Torres Strait Islander communities for the purpose of community advancement.

Initiatives such as the Maiam nayri Wingara Indigenous Data Sovereignty Collective [21] and the Indigenous Data Network (IDN) [22] have emerged as Indigenous-led groups to support the systems and governance of Indigenous data. Further, there has been a range of advocacy and negotiations between Aboriginal and Torres Strait Islander leaders and governments to further develop Indigenous data, particularly at the regional level. Recently, the IDN was funded by the Australian Government via the National Aboriginal Community Health Organisation (NACCHO), and is a part of the National Agreement on Closing the Gap [23] (National Agreement), which focuses on shared access to data and information at a regional level.

The $1.3 million project, led by Indigenous researchers and experts from around the country, was to support Priority Reform Four of the National Agreement that aims to improve and share access to data and information to enable Aboriginal and Torres Strait Islander communities to make informed decisions.

The IDN had been working in partnership with the Coalition of Aboriginal and Torres Strait Islander community-controlled peaks (Coalition of Peaks) to support the development of a new platform, which will enable Indigenous organizations to upload and analyze their own data.

"The data collected will be focused on the areas and targets, including the Priority Reforms, in the newly agreed National Agreement on Closing the Gap. It will span health, education, employment, justice, environmental management and cultural heritage services, ensuring Indigenous organisations can make evidence-based decisions to set strategies that are aligned to community needs".

"The launch of this project is the latest achievement for the IDN, which was established in 2017 to give voice to the principles of Indigenous data sovereignty—the recognition of intellectual property and other rights [24] of Indigenous people and entities in their data so that it cannot be harvested without consent by governments or any other data collector—and to lead a push for the implementation of national Indigenous data governance framework" [22].

Announcing the data project in his 2021 February address, Closing the Gap Statement to Parliament, Prime Minister Scott Morrison said that "a vital part of empowering Indigenous communities is giving them the data and information to inform their decision making." [25].

1.9. Data Sharing

The Australian government has invested significantly in its national data capabilities to monitor the progress of the nation's health through data sharing. In August 2018, the Prime Minister and Cabinet established the Office of the National Data Commissioner to build and support the infrastructure and use of public data [26]. Other national initiatives have included the National Collaborative Research Infrastructure Strategy and the Strategic Committee for National Health Information to make better use of research and health data [27]. These initiatives are developments arising from a range of internal government developments in data sharing. This includes the ABS Multi-Agency Data Integration Project (MADIP) in 2015. After its establishment, almost $131 million was invested in the Data Integration Partnership for Australia (DIPA) from 2017 to 2020 to improve technical data infrastructure and data integration capabilities across the Australian Public Service. These data assets have and continue to be used for a range of government projects and have the potential to improve statistical understandings as well as data quality.

For Aboriginal and Torres Strait Islander people there are limited mechanisms to govern Indigenous data within governments. There is currently no available information regarding who is making decisions regarding linked Aboriginal and Torres Strait Islander data and the above-mentioned data assets. In terms of data sharing, there is still a way to go regarding the interoperability of the data systems and platforms outside of government. This includes the linkage of primary health care, disease registries, and surveillance systems, and broader sectors of data collections, such as education and justice, which can provide critical insights to the distribution and determinants of health and disease in Australia.

1.10. International Indigenous Information Developments

The International Group for Indigenous Health Measurement [28] (IGIHM) was founded in 2005 and brings together Indigenous and non-Indigenous, government and non-government, statisticians, researchers, and health professionals from the four founding members of this group, Australia, Canada, New Zealand, and the United States, and, more recently, representatives from Sami organizations and Indigenous peoples from South America. The IGIHM's goals are "first, to promote awareness of the deficiencies of health data for Indigenous populations in our four countries and second, to collaborate internationally on improved methods and policies that will contribute to the improvement of Indigenous health. Since its founding in 2005, the IGIHM has pursued a variety of activities to further its goals. These activities have centred on multi-national partnerships as well as the promotion of improved methods for the collection, analysis, interpretation and dissemination of information useful for improving the health of Indigenous populations, enhancing Indigenous health knowledge and data, and the elimination of health disparities" [29]. A major recent focus has been on promoting Indigenous measurement issues in international forums including UN Statistical agencies, and the International Association for Official Statistics.

2. Pitfalls

2.1. Census

In the 1967 Referendum, Australians voted overwhelmingly to amend the Constitution to allow the Commonwealth to make laws for Aboriginal people and include them in the census. "Turnout for the referendum was almost 94 per cent, and the result was a strong 'Yes' vote, with a significant majority in all six states and an overall majority of almost 91 per cent ... " [30]. The legislation for the referendum was passed unanimously by the parliament.

The ABS had compiled experimental life tables for Indigenous Australians following the 1996 and 2001 Censuses of Population and Housing. Those estimates were compiled using different indirect demographic methods and were subject to a range of caveats [31]. Subsequently, ABS changed its methodology to direct methods. This change in method was generally welcomed although it was argued that the direct method understated Indigenous deaths and overstated life expectancy [32].

The direct method attempts to correct for under identification of deaths by use of the Post-Enumeration Survey (PES), but there is some uncertainty about the accuracy of national estimates for Indigenous life expectancy as the PES may be too small in the 60+ group, leading to high raising fractions based on small numbers of deaths, and there is also uncertainty about the adequacy of the size of the linked deaths/census sample itself. Further, the fact that ABS and AIHW produce similar estimates for life expectancy using different methods, rather than adding weight to the accuracy of both, suggests that both may overstate life expectancy as the AIHW method [33] is based on data sources, all of which are known to be incomplete.

Apart from the concerns about the accuracy of national estimates of Indigenous life expectancy derived from the census, the capacity to detect differences between successive five-yearly national life expectancy estimates, as statistically significant is at best doubtful [34]. This is in part because of significant changes in Indigenous identification between successive censuses. It is estimated that between 2011 and 2016 approximately 120,000 people who identified as non-Indigenous in 2011 identified as Indigenous in 2016, and approximately 40,000 people who identified as Indigenous in 2011 identified as non-Indigenous in 2016 [35]. Thus, a net 80,000 people changed identification from non-Indigenous to Indigenous from a census count of approximately 650,000 in 2016 and these newly identified people largely lived in cities and were better educated, more likely to be employed and had higher incomes—and were presumably healthier. Given the potential errors in each census and the proportionate size of the change in identification (approximately one in 8) and the fact that the newly identified people may well have been healthier, it becomes difficult if not impossible to determine whether any apparent increase in life expectancy between successive censuses is real or at least partially due to statistical artefact.

2.2. Backcasting

The other main method in assessing the extent of mortality or other changes over time is by the use of backcasting. "This technique requires assumptions to be made about past levels of mortality taking into account the most recent 2016 census data to utilise the best quality estimates available. These are applied to the 2016 base population to obtain a 'reverse-survived' population for the previous year. The assumptions are then applied to this new reverse-survived population to obtain a population for the preceding year. This process is repeated until the first year of the estimation period is reached [36]." ABS provides backcast population estimates for 2006–2015, but advises caution in backcasting for earlier periods:

"ABS advises that the 2001 to 2005 estimates included in the spreadsheet attached to this release should be used with caution.

Reliable life expectancy estimates of the Aboriginal and Torres Strait Islander population are not available for the period 2001 to 2005. Therefore, mortality assumptions for these years were based on trends in life expectancy during 2005–2007 and 2015–2017. There will be a greater alignment between this assumption-based mortality and the actual mortality for the years closer to the base year than those for the out years.

Moreover, estimates of the Aboriginal and Torres Strait Islander population on 30 June 2016 (based on the 2016 census) are 19% larger than those on 30 June 2011 (based on the 2011 Census). As a consequence, the use of this 2016 ERP base introduces uncertainty to the historical estimates. The uncertainty increases as the time from the base year increases".

Apart from the historical uncertainty about population estimates for earlier periods as noted by the ABS, there is a troubling circularity in the method in that in estimating trends in mortality, the method is dependent on assumptions about the mortality trends—the very parameter being estimated.

Nonetheless, government agencies show mortality trend graphs going as far back as 1998 [17,18,37]. A typical graph is shown below [18] (Figure 1). The commentary accompanying the graph says that "these changes resulted in the gap between the two populations decreasing significantly by 49% from 1998 to 2018. Most of this improvement was seen between 1998 and 2006, when the gap narrowed significantly by 42%. Over the period 2006 to 2018, the gap continued to narrow by 8% but this was not a significant change."

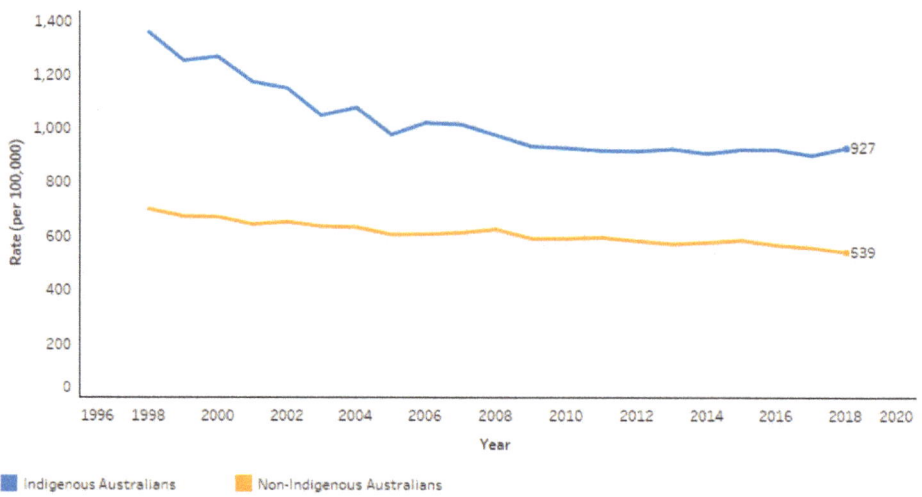

Figure 1. Age-standardized death rates, by Indigenous status, NSW, Qld, WA, SA, and NT, 1998–2018. Source: https://www.indigenoushpf.gov.au/measures/1-22-all-causes-age-standardised-death-rates. (accessed on 16 August 2021).

It is hard, if not impossible, to explain what health service, social, economic, or political changes might plausibly account for such dramatic improvements (42%) in the mortality gap between 1998 and 2006, and at the same time for a non-significant change in the mortality gap between 2006 and 2018. It is quite possible, and perhaps likely, that the apparent dramatic improvements between 1998 and 2006 were statistical artefacts associated with a lack of attention to the ABS cautionary advice, rather than real changes.

It might reasonably be concluded that it is unsafe to backcast for longer than 10 years. On that basis, the AIHW conclusion is that, "Consistent with the observed decline in mortality, life expectancy at birth increased for both Indigenous males and females during the reference period (2001–2005 to 2011–2015). However, greater increases in life expectancy at birth occurred for non-Indigenous males and females, meaning that the gap in life expectancy between Indigenous and non-Indigenous Australians widened during the reference period" [33]. This conclusion may provide the most reliable view of trends in life expectancy in recent years.

2.3. Misleading Use of Statistics

In addition to the technical issues outlined above, the most recent example of misleading use of statistics can be found in the Productivity Commission's 2021 Closing the Gap report [38].

The text here and elsewhere in the report says that this indicator (healthy birthweight) is "on track". This is manifestly not the case and is apparently based on just two points, 2017 and 2018. Projecting a trend from two points is simply inappropriate as the accompanying graph and supporting tables makes clear and the caveat does not deal with the real issue—the indicator is actually not on track. Many readers may struggle to reconcile the graph, and the commentary below it (Figure 2), indicating that there has been no change in the indicator, nationally or for any of the jurisdictions, with the assertion that the indicator is on track. A reasonable commentary based on the available information might have read, "There is insufficient data since the baseline year (2017) on which to base a trend, but the period from 2014 to 2018 does not suggest the target is on track."

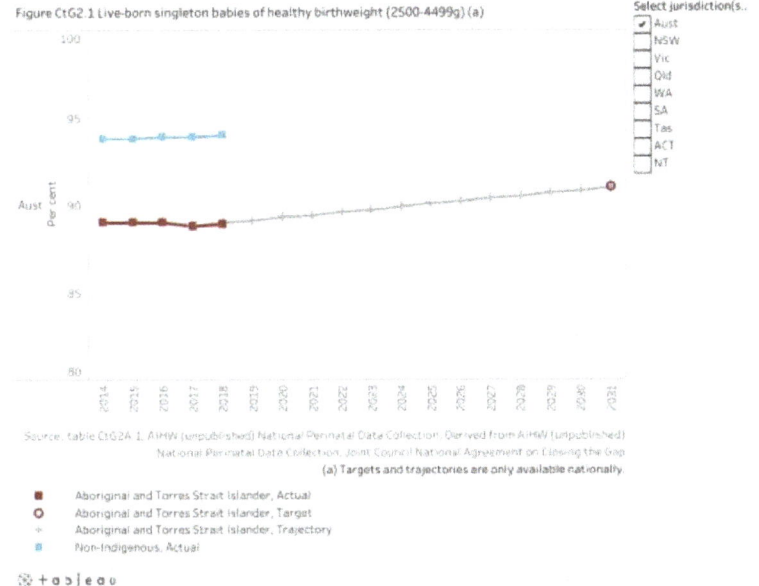

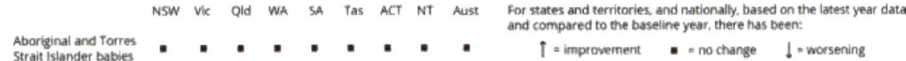

Figure 2. By 2031, increase the proportion of Aboriginal and Torres Strait Islander babies with a healthy birthweight to 91 percent. Nationally in 2018, 88.9 percent of Aboriginal and Torres Strait Islander babies born were of a healthy birthweight. This is similar to 2017 (the baseline year). Source: https://www.pc.gov.au/closing-the-gap-data/annual-data-report/2021/closing-the-gap-annual-data-compilation-report-july2021.pdf (accessed on 16 August 2021).

The interests of First Nations peoples are in no way served by asserting that such a key indicator is on track and hence current efforts to improve the health of mothers and infants are adequate, when, in reality, that is far from being the case and significantly greater effort is required so that this key indicator will cease to flatline and will start to move in the right direction. The material from the report for this indicator is shown above.

2.4. Use of Information

Though there were and are limitations in the data that were available and some significant gaps in available information, for many years now, there has been a wealth of information that was available and readily accessible to administrators and policy makers. The Aboriginal and Torres Strait Islander Health Performance Framework, the Health and Welfare of Australia's Aboriginal and Torres Strait Islander Peoples, the OID Reports, and the annual Closing the Gap Reports released by the Prime Minister at the opening of parliament each year all provide a wealth of information on health indices and progress or lack of progress.

Yet there seems no formal process for policy makers and service providers to examine each report and take policy and management decisions on the findings. The process seems little better than sitting around hoping next year's numbers might look better without taking formal action to evaluate the findings and take the necessary action to improve performance—particularly in a climate where all can see that progress has been inadequate. This is in part because: evaluation is generally bitty, piecemeal, and not embedded in a formal policy and planning cycle; in part because the sheer volume of material makes it almost indigestible; a false sense of reassurance compounded by misrepresentation of statistical artefact as real progress; too little information is available on the availability of, funding for, access to, appropriateness or effectiveness of services required to improve outcomes; also because indicators are reported on as discrete measures separately and independently and the interrelationship between them not specified (if progress in all causes mortality is disappointing, no information is provided on services for chronic disease); information is generally only available at national and jurisdictional levels rather than service delivery or community levels; but above all there is simply no formal process to examine the content of these reports and see what lessons could and should be learnt to achieve the progress specified in national goals.

Monthly, six monthly, and annual reviews to examine available data on performance are not a feature at any level, certainly not at national, jurisdictional, or regional levels, though some services may be doing so. This is amateur hour writ large—and the consequences for the health and welfare of Aboriginal and Torres Strait Islander people are very significant in terms of preventable admissions and deaths.

2.5. Surveillance and Monitoring Services

There is a pressing need to ensure that disease surveillance systems and service monitoring continue to be efficient, effective, and appropriate to enable timely and appropriate services to the public. This includes communicable and non-communicable diseases as well as primary health care services. Perhaps the most immediate issue impacting Aboriginal and Torres Strait Islander people is the absence of the Indigenous identifier on private pathology request forms. This affects measurement of many issues, cancer, infectious diseases, and currently COVID-19. When knowledge of testing rates is so critical to the prevention and management of COVID-19 and with Indigenous people at particular risk, it is hard to believe that this most crucial piece of information is still lacking despite numerous calls for improvement. Most recently, the National Aboriginal and Torres Strait Islander COVID-19 Management Plan [39] had the recommendation for a remit to improve data collection and Aboriginal and Torres Strait Islander identification in healthcare and pathology testing.

More generally, notwithstanding the 1994 AHMAC decision that the highest national health information priority was to "work with Aboriginal and Torres Strait Islander peoples to develop a plan to improve all aspects of information about their health and health services [6]", most of the subsequent development work on Indigenous health information has centred around health rather than health services, although AIHW has done some useful work in this area [40,41] and the HPF and the OID Reports provide some basic information. Nonetheless, there is little essential information available on service gaps (which could, for example, be defined as areas with high levels of preventable admissions and deaths and low use of the Medical and Pharmaceutical Benefits Schedules BMBS/PBS) and less about how well services that do exist actually work. The Productivity Commission found that, "There are many Australian Government policies and programs that are designed to improve the lives of Aboriginal and Torres Strait Islander people. But after decades of developing new policies and programs and modifying existing ones, we still know very little about their impact on Aboriginal and Torres Strait Islander people, or how outcomes could be improved [42]." This has been a serious omission as it has meant that much information has been provided about health issues for Aboriginal and Torres Strait Islander peoples, but not the kind of information which would provide policy makers and administrators with the information required for more effective action to address those health issues.

3. Prospects

3.1. Life Expectancy

Progress with some of the issues outlined above is certainly possible. While attempting to estimate changes in life expectancy from successive censuses is unsafe and backcasting population estimates beyond 10 years produces unreliable and implausible results, it is likely that estimating changes in life expectancy within a 10-year period using backcast population estimates, as carried out by AIHW [33] can provide a useable estimate of trend, even though the levels of life expectancy may be overestimated through the use of data sources each of which is known to under identify Indigenous people.

To its credit, the ABS commissioned an independent review of its Indigenous life expectancy estimate in 2019, which reported in 2021.

Taylor and her colleagues [34] seem to favour the cohort-interpolated approach over the backcasting method for estimating populations and that warrants further investigation. Equally, the Voluntary Indigenous Identifier (VII) on Medicare data may be sufficiently complete to provide an alternative source of identification and it may be appropriate for both ABS and AIHW to consider the potential for using the VII as a tool to reduce under identification in death records.

3.2. Identifiers on Private Pathology Request Forms

This issue has been on the national agenda for years but remains unresolved. Similar issues on the inclusion of indigenous identifiers on the records of private hospitals were dealt with decades ago and COVID-19 provides a real opportunity for the issue to be finally rectified along the lines recommended in the 2013 AIHW Report [43].

3.3. Community Level Data

"Accurate and locally relevant data on demographics, health outcomes, health determinants and access to services is key to inform decision making by local communities, services and for program and policy evaluations [44]." However, provision of data at small area level presents significant, technical and logistical challenges. The AIHW is developing an Indigenous Community Insights website which will facilitate access to data at a regional level and also produces data for Indigenous Advancement Strategy (IAS) regions and sub regions. The IDN is also focused on provision of regional level data and as Professor Langton said, "By supporting communities and community-controlled organisations to collect their own data and use government-held data, the coalition of peaks and the IDN are helping communities to tell their own stories about what is working for them and what isn't [22]".

3.4. Measuring Wellbeing

"Accurate wellbeing measures tell us what works and what does not work to improve wellbeing, inform patient and clinical decision making, service delivery, policy, and ultimately improve patient outcomes. The absence of a robust culturally relevant wellbeing measure has significantly hindered progress in improving wellbeing for all Aboriginal and

Torres Strait Islander Australians" [45]. This topic is of interest and importance both nationally and internationally [46–50]. Within Australia, Professor Garvey and her colleagues have developed and are testing a nationally relevant instrument to measure the wellbeing of Aboriginal and Torres Strait adults. The measure includes 32 items across 10 dimensions including, for example: Balance and Control, Hope and Resilience, Culture and Country, Spirit and Identity, and Racism and Worries. The research team are developing a short form version of What Matters 2 Adults and have commenced work to develop a What Matters 2 youth wellbeing measure (12–17 years) and are piloting a project to test methods with Aboriginal and Torres Strait Islander children <11 years [46].

3.5. Use of Data for Management Purposes

The ground-breaking new National Agreement on Closing the Gap between the Coalition of Aboriginal and Torres Strait Islander Peak Organisations and all Australian governments [23] provides for "Shared access to location specific data and information [that] will support Aboriginal and Torres Strait Islander communities and organisations to support the achievement of the Priority Reforms" through partnership, "making evidence-based decisions on the design, implementation and evaluation of policies and programs for their communities in order to develop local solutions for local issues and "measuring the transformation of government organisations operating in their region to be more responsive and accountable for Closing the Gap". There is also an acceptance of the desirability of local level data to enable local decision-making, and the need for Aboriginal and Torres Strait Islander communities and organisations to be "supported by governments to build capability and expertise in collecting, using and interpreting data in a meaningful way".

If translated into action, these agreements would be very important reforms. However, they will not necessarily resolve the fundamental issue, of not just guaranteeing access to data, but using that data at all levels of government, by service providers to improve performance. The failure to fully utilize the data that does exist is a central element in the relative lack of progress in recent years. This is because access to and provision of data is not an end in itself, but an integral element in the policy and planning cycle, where data is used to monitor and improve performance, refine policy, and progressively improve outcomes as set out in the Planning Cycle diagram [51] below (Figure 3).

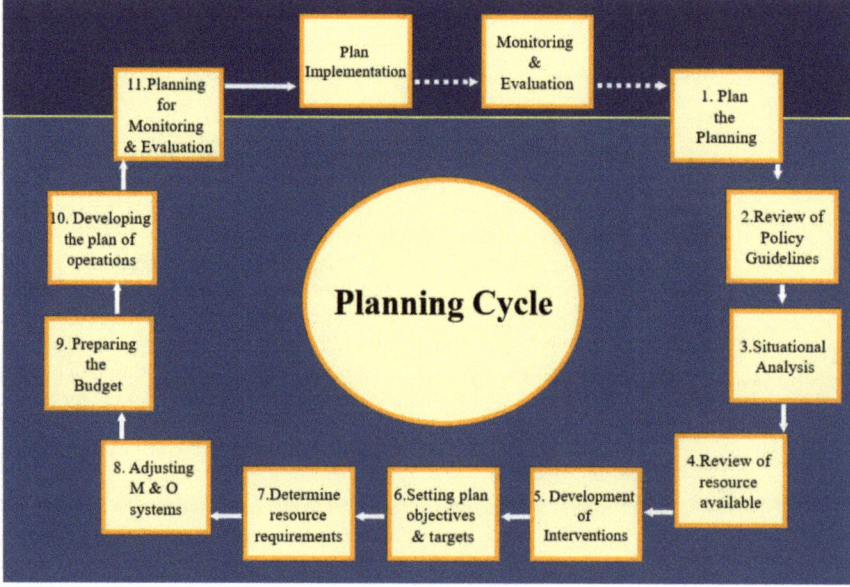

Figure 3. Planning Cycle.

Information should play a vital role in several of the Actions in the Planning Cycle diagram—in Step 3, Situational Analysis; in Step 4, Review of available resources; and most importantly in Monitoring and Evaluation in Step 11, but at present is not being utilised to anything like its full potential [52–57]. Note also that the cycle is just that, a continuous cycle, not a static or periodic process. An essential requirement is to have formal reviews of performance at monthly intervals for service providers, and six monthly and annual reviews involving communities, funders, service providers, and policy makers.

3.6. Indigenous Data Governance

There are still many issues that need to be resolved regarding Aboriginal and Torres Strait Islander data in official statistics. Despite the investments in data capabilities in Australia, efforts are still needed to meet the needs and aspirations of Aboriginal and Torres Strait Islander people by facilitating Indigenous Data Sovereignty through Indigenous Data Governance processes. One recommendation is that Aboriginal and Torres Strait Islander people are supported in the development of mechanisms to govern their data. This should be in alignment with current developments in ID-SOV, whereby Indigenous peoples have the right to exercise authority and govern the affairs of the use of Indigenous data that reflects Indigenous peoples interests and aspirations [58]. For Aboriginal and Torres Strait Islander people, this is enacting self-determination in the collection and use of data and acts to redress the existing unequal power distributions currently seen in Australian society. It is important to ensure that Aboriginal and Torres Strait Islander epidemiologists and demographers lead the way in discussions on data collection, quality, and reporting regarding official statistics. This is to enable existing data infrastructures and data systems to work optimally for Aboriginal and Torres Strait Islander people and to ensure there are established mechanisms of expert voice as Aboriginal and Torres Strait Islander communities move closer towards data control and ownership within Australia.

4. Conclusions

Much progress has been made in the provision of information but there are a number of immediate challenges—and opportunities. A central lesson of the past is that for information to achieve its potential, it has to be used and used in a way which links policy, funding, implementation, monitoring and evaluation in a continuous policy/planning cycle, and that cycle has yet to be instituted in a systematic way across all levels of service delivery, government and communities. There is now the potential for Aboriginal and Torres Strait Islanders to be not just partners but leaders in the design, collection and use of information, but this also requires a concerted effort to train Aboriginal and Torres Strait Islanders for those tasks and responsibilities.

Author Contributions: Conceptualization, I.R.; methodology, I.R., K.G.; writing—original draft preparation, I.R., K.G.; writing—review and editing, I.R., K.G. All authors have read and agreed to the published version of the manuscript.

Funding: This research received no external funding.

Institutional Review Board Statement: Not applicable.

Informed Consent Statement: Not applicable.

Data Availability Statement: Not applicable.

Conflicts of Interest: The authors declare no conflict of interest.

References

1. Thompson, N. An historical overview of the development of Indigenous Health Statistics. Indigenous Identification in Administrative Data Collections: Best Practice and Quality Assurance. In *Report on Workshop Proceedings, November 1996*; ABS & AIHW, Commonwealth of Australia: Canberra, Australia, 1997.
2. Smith, L.R. *Aboriginal Health Statistics in Australia—A Survey and a Plan*, 3rd ed.; Health Research Group, Australian National University: Canberra, Australia, 1978.

3. Griffiths, K.; Coleman, C.; Al-Yaman, F.; Cunningham, J.; Garvey, G.; Whop, L.; Pulver, J.L.; Ring, I.; Madden, R. The identification of Aboriginal and Torres Strait Islander people in official statistics and other data: Critical issues of international significance. *JIAOS* **2019**, *35*, 91–106. [CrossRef]
4. AIHW. *The Health and Welfare of Australia's Aboriginal and Torres Strait Is Lander Peoples*; AIHW: Canberra, Australia, 1997; AIHW Cat. no. IHW 2, ABS Cat. no. 4704.0.
5. Available online: https://www.aihw.gov.au/getmedia/022ad693-20a7-4ccf-a816-d338453ca46a/HWI-6-NHWI-News-7.pdf.aspx?inline=true (accessed on 16 August 2021).
6. AIHW. *The Aboriginal and Torres Strait Islander Health Information Plan: This Time, Let's Make It Happen*; AIHW: Canberra, Australia, 1997; AIHW Cat. no. IHW 12.
7. ABS. *National Aboriginal and Torres Strait Island Survey 4190.0*; ABS: Canberra, Australia, 1994.
8. Available online: http://www.austlii.edu.au/au/other/IndigLRes/rciadic/national/vol5/5.html (accessed on 16 August 2021).
9. AIHW. *National Advisory Group on Aboriginal and Torres Strait Islander Health Information and Data: Strategic Plan 2010–2015*; Cat. No. IHW 57. IHW; Australian Institute of Health and Welfare (AIHW): Canberra, Australia, 2011.
10. AIHW. *NAGATSIHID Strategic Plan 2006–2008*; AIHW: Canberra, Australia, 2006; Cat no IHW 19.
11. Available online: https://www.abs.gov.au/about/aboriginal-and-torres-strait-islander-peoples/aboriginal-and-torres-strait-islander-engagement#the-round-table-on-aboriginal-and-torres-strait-islander-statistics (accessed on 22 September 2021).
12. AIHW Indigenous Statistical and Information Advisory group; (Canberra, Australia). Personal Communication, 2021.
13. Available online: https://www.abs.gov.au/ausstats/abs@.nsf/DOSSbyTopic/1A8650F3AF9F5C70CA256BD00028807F?OpenDocument (accessed on 16 August 2021).
14. Vines, A.P. *An Epidemiological Sample Survey of the Highlands, Mainland and Islands Regions of the Territory of Paua and New Guinea*; Department of Public Health: Port Moresby, Papua New Guinea, 1970.
15. Australain Bureau of Statistics (ABS). *Australian Aboriginal and Torres Strait Islander Health Survey: Biomedical Results, 2012–2013*; Edith Cowan University: Perth, Australia, 2014; ABS 4727.0.55.003.
16. Available online: https://www.pc.gov.au/research/ongoing/overcoming-indigenous-disadvantage (accessed on 16 August 2021).
17. SCRGSP (Steering Committee for the Review of Government Service Provision). *Overcoming Indigenous Disadvantage: Key Indicators 2020*; Productivity Commission: Canberra, Australia, 2020.
18. Australian Institute of Health and Welfare. *Aboriginal and Torres Strait Islander Health Performance Framework 2020 Summary Report*; AIHW: Canberra, Australia, 2020; Cat. no. IHPF 2.
19. Steering Committee for the Review of Government Service Provision. *2017 Indigenous Expenditure Report*; Productivity Commission: Canberra, Australia, 2017.
20. Available online: https://indigenoushpf.gov.au/measures/3-21-expenditure-atsi-compared-need (accessed on 16 August 2021).
21. Available online: https://www.maiamnayriwingara.org/about-us (accessed on 16 August 2021).
22. Available online: https://about.unimelb.edu.au/newsroom/news/2020/september/$1.3-million-indigenous-data-project-to-transform-community-outcomes (accessed on 16 August 2021).
23. Available online: https://www.closingthegap.gov.au/sites/default/files/files/national-agreement-ctg.pdf (accessed on 16 August 2021).
24. Available online: https://www.un.org/development/desa/indigenouspeoples/wp-content/uploads/sites/19/2018/11/UNDRIP_E_web.pdf (accessed on 22 September 2021).
25. Available online: https://www.pm.gov.au/media/address-closing-gap-statement-parliament (accessed on 16 August 2021).
26. Australian Government. *Best Practice Guide to Applying Data Sharing Principles*; Department of Prime Minister and Cabinet: Canberra, Australia, 2019.
27. Available online: https://www.aihw.gov.au/our-services/committees/strategic-committee-for-national-health-information (accessed on 16 August 2021).
28. Available online: https://www.aihw.gov.au/our-services/international-collaboration/international-group-indigenous-health-measurement (accessed on 16 August 2021).
29. Chino, M.; Ring, I.; Pulver, L.J.; Waldon, J.; King, M. Improving health data for indigenous populations: The international group for indigenous health measurement. *Stat. J. IAOS* **2019**, *35*, 15–21. [CrossRef]
30. Available online: https://www.aph.gov.au/About_Parliament/Parliamentary_Departments/Parliamentary_Library/FlagPost/2017/May/The_1967_Referendum (accessed on 16 August 2021).
31. Australian Bureau of Statistics. *3302.0.55.002-Discussion Paper: Assessment of Methods for Developing Life Tables for Aboriginal and Torres Strait Islander Australians*; Australian Bureau of Statistics: Canberra, Australia, 2006.
32. Madden, R.; Tickle, L.; Jackson Pulver, L.; Ring, L. Estimating Indigenous life expectancy: Pitfalls with consequences. *J. Pop. Res.* **2012**, *29*, 269–281. [CrossRef]
33. Australian Institute of Health and Welfare. *Trends in Indigenous Mortality and Life Expectancy, 2001–2015: Evidence from the Enhanced Mortality Database*; Cat. no. IHW 174; AIHW: Canberra, Australia, 2017.
34. Taylor, A.; Barnes, A.; Paradies, Y. *Independent Review of the Australian Bureau of Statistics' Aboriginal and Torres Strait Islander Life Expectancy Estimates*; Australian Bureau of Statistics: Canberra, Australia, 2021; (Available on request from ABS).

35. Australian Bureau of Statistics (ABS). *Census of Population and Housing: Understanding the Increase in Aboriginal and Torres Strait Islander Counts*; Australian Bureau of Statistics: Canberra, Australia, 2018; ABS 2077.0.
36. Available online: https://www.abs.gov.au/statistics/people/aboriginal-and-torres-strait-islander-peoples/estimates-and-projections-aboriginal-and-torres-strait-islander-australians/latest-release (accessed on 16 August 2021).
37. Available online: https://ctgreport.niaa.gov.au/sites/default/files/pdf/closing-the-gap-report-2020.pdf (accessed on 16 August 2021).
38. Available online: https://www.pc.gov.au/closing-the-gap-data/annual-data-report/2021/closing-the-gap-annual-data-compilation-report-july2021.pdf (accessed on 16 August 2021).
39. Available online: https://www.health.gov.au/resources/publications/management-plan-for-aboriginal-and-torres-strait-islander-populations (accessed on 17 August 2021).
40. Australian Institute of Health and Welfare. *Spatial Variation in Aboriginal and Torres Strait Islander Women's Access to 4 Types of Maternal Health Services*; Cat. no. IHW 187; AIHW: Canberra, Australia, 2017.
41. AIHW (Australian Institute of Health and Welfare). *Access to Primary Health Care Relative to Need for Indigenous Australians*; Cat. no. IHW 128; AIHW: Canberra, Australia, 2014.
42. Productivity Commission, Indigenous Evaluation Strategy. 2020. Available online: https://www.pc.gov.au/inquiries/completed/indigenous-evaluation/strategy/indigenous-evaluation-strategy.pdf (accessed on 16 August 2021).
43. Australian Institute of Health and Welfare. *The Inclusion of Indigenous Status on Pathology Request Forms*; AIHW: Canberra, Australia, 2013; Cat. no. IHW 103.
44. Available online: https://www.pc.gov.au/__data/assets/pdf_file/0003/245451/sub099-indigenous-evaluation.pdf (accessed on 16 August 2021).
45. Available online: https://timhwb.org.au/sewb-gathering-reports/ (accessed on 16 August 2021).
46. Available online: https://indigenouswellness.ca/wp-content/uploads/2018/08/IGIHM-Indigenous-Wellness-Indicators-Day-A-Synthesis.pdf (accessed on 16 August 2021).
47. Biddle, N. Measuring and Analysing the Wellbeing of Australia's Indigenous Population. *Soc. Indic. Res.* **2014**, *116*, 713–729. [CrossRef]
48. Dockery, A.M. Culture and Wellbeing: The Case of Indigenous Australians. *Soc. Indic. Res.* **2010**, *99*, 315–332. [CrossRef]
49. Haswell, M.R.; Kavanagh, D.; Tsey, K.; Reilly, L.; Cadet-James, Y.; Laliberte, A.; Wilson, A.; Doran, C. Psychometric validation of the Growth and Empowerment Measure (GEM) applied with Indigenous Australians. *Aust. N. Z. J. Psychiatry* **2010**, *44*, 791. [CrossRef] [PubMed]
50. Manning, M.; Ambrey, C.L.; Fleming, C.M. A Longitudinal Study of Indigenous Wellbeing in Australia. *J. Happiness Stud.* **2016**, *17*, 2503–2525. [CrossRef]
51. Available online: https://www.gfmer.ch/SRH-Course-2011/Geneva-Workshop/pdf/Health-planning-cycle-Ali-2012.pdf (accessed on 16 August 2021).
52. Mashford-Pringle, A.; Ring, I.; Al-Yaman, F.; Waldon, J.; Chino, M. Rethinking health services measurement for Indigenous populations. *Stat. J. IAOS* **2019**, *35*, 139–146. [CrossRef]
53. Ring, I. Close the Gap and national health reform. *Aust. Med.* **2010**, *22*, 25–26.
54. Mathews, A.; Pulver, L.; Ring, I. How are Indigenous health policy directions formulated for chronic disease, and what can be done to strengthen the link between policy formulation and implementation? *Aust. Health Rev.* **2008**, *32*, 613–625. [CrossRef] [PubMed]
55. Ring, I.; Brown, N. Aboriginal and Torres Strait Islander Health Implementation, not more policies. *J. Aust. Indig. Issues* **2003**, *6*, 3–12.
56. Ring, I.T.; Brown, N. Indigenous Health: Chronically inadequate responses to damning statistics. *Med. J. Aust.* **2002**, *177*, 629–631. [CrossRef] [PubMed]
57. Ring, I. Editorial-A 'whole of government' approach needed on Indigenous health. *Aust. J. Public Health* **1998**, *22*, 639–640. [CrossRef] [PubMed]
58. Kukutai, T.; Taylor, J.Y. *Indigenous Data Sovereignty: Towards an Agenda, in Research Monograph 38-Centre for Aboriginal Economic Policy Research*; Kukutai, T., Taylor, J.Y., Eds.; Australian National University Press: Canberra, Australia, 2016.

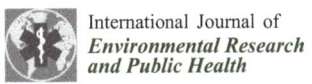

Brief Report

Enhancing Australian Mortality Data to Meet Future Health Information Demands

James Eynstone-Hinkins and Lauren Moran *

Australian Bureau of Statistics, Canberra 2616, Australia; james.eynstone-hinkins@abs.gov.au
* Correspondence: lauren.moran@abs.gov.au

Abstract: The Australian mortality data are a foundational health dataset which supports research, policy and planning. The COVID-19 pandemic necessitated the need for more timely mortality data that could assist in monitoring direct mortality from the virus as well as indirect mortality due to social and economic societal change. This paper discusses the evolution of mortality data in Australia during the pandemic and looks at emerging opportunities associated with electronic infrastructure such as electronic Medical Certificates of Cause of Death (eMCCDs), ICD-11 and automated coding tools that will form the foundations of a more responsive and comprehensive future mortality dataset.

Keywords: mortality data; cause of death; coronial investigation

Citation: Eynstone-Hinkins, J.; Moran, L. Enhancing Australian Mortality Data to Meet Future Health Information Demands. *Int. J. Environ. Res. Public Health* **2022**, *19*, 603. https://doi.org/10.3390/ijerph19010603

Academic Editor: Richard Madden

Received: 2 November 2021
Accepted: 31 December 2021
Published: 5 January 2022

Publisher's Note: MDPI stays neutral with regard to jurisdictional claims in published maps and institutional affiliations.

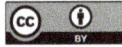

Copyright: © 2022 by the authors. Licensee MDPI, Basel, Switzerland. This article is an open access article distributed under the terms and conditions of the Creative Commons Attribution (CC BY) license (https:// creativecommons.org/licenses/by/ 4.0/).

1. Introduction

The national mortality dataset (NMD) in Australia is produced annually by the Australian Bureau of Statistics (ABS). Data are sourced from the civil registration and vital statistics system, and provide a foundation for both population and heath research, policy and planning. As life expectancy has increased over the past century, the NMD has charted key changes in population health which have contributed to these gains. Key changes include large reductions in infant mortality rates [1], decreases in coronary artery disease mortality since 1968 [2], the aging of the population and the subsequent emergence of dementia as a leading cause of death [3].

The NMD has evolved and improved significantly over its long history. Many improvements are related to enhancements to the death registration process, with more thorough death investigation processes and recording of key demographic details leading to improvements in source data. Advancements in medical science and technology have led to improved diagnosis of diseases and cause of death certification. As knowledge about diseases and death has improved, the classification that underpins mortality data—the International Classification of Diseases (ICD)—has also been revised, leading to incremental changes in mortality datasets over time.

The NMD is part of a rich tapestry of health information data in Australia and has been more commonly used for epidemiological research and annual tracking of patterns of death. Health surveillance systems have produced rapid data for certain causes such as influenza, providing policy makers with timely information that can direct intervention and prevention activities when required. Health surveillance systems have also played the primary role in monitoring mortality due to COVID-19 during the pandemic.

As the COVID-19 pandemic has progressed there has been growing recognition of the importance of Civil Registration and Vital Statistics (CRVS) systems in filling key data gaps, as governments seek to understand its full impact on population health. Measures of excess mortality (the numbers of deaths that occur during a defined period compared to the number of expected deaths during that same period) help track both direct COVID-19 mortality and indirect mortality, for instance deaths which might relate to changes in access to health care [4]. In mid-2020 the ABS began releasing provisional mortality reports. These reports focused on all deaths that were doctor certified, and provided early indications of changes in patterns of mortality, including excess deaths, for key causes.

The demand for rapid mortality information continues to be driven by subsequent waves of COVID-19 and recognition that the longer-term effects of the pandemic need to be identified and addressed as early as possible. This is driving innovation in the way data is collected, analysed and used. This paper focuses on recent initiatives aimed at enhancing the NMD, and emerging opportunities associated with new electronic infrastructure that could shape the next generation of both health and mortality data.

2. Current Mortality Dataset Foundations

State and territory Registries of Births, Deaths and Marriages (RBDMs) are legislatively responsible for death registration in Australia. There are minor differences in form design and variables collected across jurisdictions, but the death registration process is generally consistent across the country. Death registrations require both a death registration statement (DRS) completed by an informant with the funeral director, and a medical certificate cause of death (MCCD) completed by a doctor. The format of the MCCD is based on the standard recommended by the World Health Organization. RBDMs lodge complete death registrations with the ABS for the compilation of the NMD.

Approximately 12% of deaths in Australia are referred to a coroner. While a death referred to a coroner must still follow the death registration process governed by the jurisdictional RBDMs, information pertaining to the cause of death is stored in the National Coronial Information System (NCIS). The NCIS is a medico-legal online database that holds information pertaining to coroner-referred deaths including police, toxicology, pathology and coronial reports [5]. This information is accessed by the ABS for coding of causes of death.

The DRS is used to inform the demographic component of mortality data with the cause of death coming from the MCCD or the NCIS. Cause of death certification is of high quality, with Australia found to have the lowest proportion of 'unusable' causes of death in a recent study focused on six high resource countries [6].

Australian cause of death information is coded using the 10th revision of the International Classification of Diseases (ICD-10). The automated coding system, Iris, is used assist with ICD-10 coding. Iris assigns ICD-10 codes to all terms on death certificates, then applies coding rules to select the underlying cause of death (the disease or condition that initiated the train of morbid events leading to death). Manual coding is required for most coroner referred deaths and doctor certified records unable to be processed by Iris.

Enhancements to the NMD are ongoing and target both demographic and cause of death variables. Enhancements to the demographic component are prioritised to support government priorities. The quality of identification of Aboriginal and Torres Strait Islander people on death registration documents is a high priority and has been a focus for both the ABS and RBDMs. More recently, place of death information was highlighted as a priority, with a framework subsequently developed to classify and capture this information [7].

Cause of death coding and output is also subject to frequent improvements. Since 1997, coded information on all causes listed on the death certificate (multiple cause data) has been retained. Multiple cause data provides important insights into the complex nature of death which has increasing relevance with an ageing population and people living with multiple co-morbidities which may collectively cause many pathways to death. This dataset is progressively being used to greater effect as methods for multiple cause analysis are strengthened, providing insights into relationships between diseases and their relative contributions to mortality.

Coronial investigative reports on the NCIS provide a rich source of information on circumstances and causes of coroner referred deaths. Risk factors for coroner referred deaths which are not a diagnosable disease but may have a detrimental impact on health are now coded as part of the NMD using ICD frameworks. Common risk factors relating to suicide deaths include previous self-harm attempts, disruption of family by separation or divorce, problems relating to economic or legal circumstances, unemployment and homelessness. Risk factors also vary with age, highlighting the importance of chronic health conditions and limitations to activity as key factors among older age groups [8].

Rapid Reporting during the COVID-19 Pandemic

The COVID-19 pandemic created a demand for accurate and timely information on causes of death. The health surveillance system in Australia can provide rapid updates on COVID-19 mortality, but data only includes numbers of deaths and key demographics. It was recognized early in the pandemic that CRVS-based data would be able to provide important additional insights. Multiple cause data could provide insights into common comorbidities and consequences of the virus, while monitoring patterns of deaths across all causes could give insights into indirect effects of the pandemic or undiagnosed COVID-19 deaths.

There were challenges that needed to be addressed to enable rapid provision of CRVS-based mortality data during the pandemic. ICD coding challenges included the application of new rules for coding COVID-19 related deaths (rules were released by WHO in April 2020 and applied to all deaths where COVID-19 was mentioned on death certificates) and fast-tracking coding of all other deaths. Another key challenge was enabling meaningful comparison of rapid data against historical data. Investigations into issues of timeliness and completeness of data were conducted and guided key decisions on data releases.

In Australia, the time between when a death occurs and data lodgement is affected by the legislative requirement for burial or cremation prior to registration. While most doctor-certified deaths are registered within one month, it can be longer if the period between death and burial or cremation is prolonged. This period can be longer for coroner-referred deaths depending on circumstances and requirements of the coronial investigation.

System limitations necessitated scope changes for the production of the monthly NMD. These monthly outputs report on doctor-certified deaths only. The time between death and registration is shorter for doctor-certified deaths so more complete data is able to be published more rapidly. Data is also published by date of death to accurately measure mortality temporal to the pandemic. This differs to normal vital statistics reporting which is usually based on numbers of death registrations received in a specified period. Rapid data must be representative of the period of interest to enable meaningful comparison. Data in the monthly report is also considered to be provisional. This allows for deaths which are registered at a later time to be added once received [9].

Monthly provisional datasets use crude measures to highlight potential changes in patterns of mortality. A five-year average of raw counts of deaths is used as a proxy to measure expected deaths, with minimum and maximum numbers of deaths over that period provided to indicate a possible range. This method is applied to deaths from all causes and to specified causes of death. Age-standardised death rates with corresponding confidence intervals are also published to enable measurement of change over time.

Official calculations of excess mortality applied a robust regression to produce an expected number of deaths for 2020 [10]. Prediction intervals of 95% were also calculated. Only deaths which exceeded the upper bound of the prediction interval were considered to be excess. While excess mortality was recorded in some weeks, this was not sustained and, overall, during 2020, Australia did not record excess mortality. In the winter months, lower than expected mortality was recorded with the reduction reaching statistical significance. Measures in place to prevent the spread of COVID-19 likely led to a reduction in deaths from other causes, especially respiratory diseases. Similar patterns of mortality during the pandemic have been reported in New Zealand, Denmark and Norway [11].

COVID-19 has raised awareness of the importance of civil registration based mortality data in many countries, also leading to enhanced cooperation between agencies and accelerating the digitisation of registration services [12]. In Australia, it has driven a need to re-think some aspects of mortality data collection and reporting, highlighting new opportunities to further enhance the timeliness and relevance future datasets.

3. New Electronic Foundations for Mortality Data Systems

The COVID-19 pandemic has reinforced the importance of CRVS-based mortality data for both epidemiological study and for monitoring emerging public health concerns. Delivering on COVID-19 related data needs has helped identify barriers to rapid data production across the CRVS system, also highlighting where changes could result in significant improvements. In Australia, the delay between when deaths occur and when they are registered, time required to quality assure data and the complexity of cause of death coding, all contribute to delays in data availability.

The electronic transformation of the CRVS system provides an opportunity to streamline and further automate production of the NMD. In particular, the implementation of electronic Medical Certificates of Cause of Death (eMCCDs), the adoption of ICD-11 and the development and implementation of next generation auto-coding systems hold great potential to overcome existing system limitations.

3.1. Electronic Medical Certificates of Cause of Death

A key component of the electronic transformation of the CRVS system is the development of eMCCDs. These electronic forms have been developed by many countries and offer key advantages to paper forms. The instant digital capture of information supplied by a medical practitioner will reduce the time between when a death occurs and when information on that death can be made available. Electronic data capture also removes the need for transcription, improving timeliness and accuracy by eliminating transcription errors.

Early versions of eMCCDs in Australia follow similar formats to paper forms, but opportunities exist to enhance these products into the future. Electronic forms could improve the quality of certification by flagging sequencing errors or requesting additional information from the certifier. These forms could also link to the ICD foundations, potentially reducing error in data capture and enabling some degree of automated coding to occur during data collection.

3.2. ICD-11

The 11th revision of the ICD was adopted by the World Health Assembly in 2019 and is now available for implementation. ICD-11 was designed as an electronic classification. All entities including diseases, disorders, injuries and symptoms are stored in the ICD-11 foundation with each defined in a standard way using a structured content model. All entities also have their own URI, with a web-service API enabling direct links to other electronic infrastructure and health information systems [13]. These new capabilities go beyond the usual advancements in medical and scientific knowledge associated with an ICD revision and will make the classification a more integrated part of future health information infrastructure.

ICD-11 also enables capture of additional information about diseases and conditions using extension codes. In the mortality use case, extension codes may capture additional information on non-proprietary names of drugs for drug related deaths, or risk factors for external cause deaths. The possibilities associated with extension codes are extensive and may only be limited by the information available when coding and compiling data. Concepts such as post-coordination and clustering of codes have been proposed to provide structure to more complex ICD-11 datasets, although methods for structuring and using groups of codes will need further consideration.

3.3. Automated Coding Solutions

Auto-coding systems are critical for processing the large number of deaths that occur in Australia, allowing codes to be assigned to individual entities and automated rules to be applied for the selection of underlying causes of death. Australia uses the Iris mortality auto-coding system, with this product enabling auto-coding of around 65% of doctor certified deaths each year. A project is now underway to develop an ICD-11 version of Iris. This project seeks to realise the benefits of the extended vocabulary and concepts of ICD-11, to integrate with ICD-11 tools, to interface with healthcare systems and eMCCDs and use advanced techniques such as machine leaning to detect certification errors and increase auto-coding rates [14].

The new electronic components of the CRVS system hold the key to transforming information from death certificates into usable epidemiological data in a way that is rapid, automated, reliable and accurate, and consistent across institutions and countries [14], and will ensure mortality data can meet future information demands including those highlighted by COVID-19.

4. Conclusions

CRVS-based mortality datasets, including Australia's NMD, are important epidemiological datasets that have guided health policy and planning for many years. The COVID-19 pandemic has highlighted the importance of rapid reporting of CRVS-based mortality data to complement data collected through surveillance systems and provide insights into the broader impacts of the pandemic beyond deaths directly from the virus.

Work undertaken in Australia to provide rapid data during the pandemic highlighted systemwide limitations that narrowed the scope of reported data. In particular, reporting needed to be sufficiently lagged to enable meaningful interpretation of changes in mortality, and only doctor-certified deaths could be included in reports. This limited the types of policy questions that could be addressed through rapid reporting to those concerning deaths from natural causes.

In Australia, electronic foundations already exist within the CRVS system with additional electronic components being developed and implemented by jurisdictional RBDMs. The electronic transformation of the CRVS system is expanding opportunities, with eMCCDs, ICD-11 and next-generation auto-coding tools likely to streamline future data collection, processing and reporting.

While COVID-19 has provided a catalyst for innovation and set clear new requirements for CRVS-based mortality datasets, the potential uses of rapid mortality data extend well beyond the pandemic. Rapid data will be able to provide early indications of changes in patterns of mortality relating to any number of events that could impact population health, including natural disasters, changes in natural cause patterns of mortality or infectious-disease-related epidemics.

Author Contributions: Writing—original draft preparation, J.E.-H., L.M.; writing—review and editing, J.E.-H., L.M. All authors have read and agreed to the published version of the manuscript.

Funding: This research received no external funding.

Institutional Review Board Statement: Not applicable.

Informed Consent Statement: Not applicable.

Data Availability Statement: Not applicable.

Conflicts of Interest: The authors declare no conflict of interest.

References

1. Australian Bureau of Statistics. *Life Tables, States, Territories and Australia, 2014–2016, Life Expectancy Improvements over the Last 125 Years*; ABS Cat; Australian Bureau of Statistics: Canberra, Australia, 2017.
2. Australian Bureau of Statistics. *Changing Patterns of Mortality in Australia, 2018*; Australian Bureau of Statistics: Canberra, Australia, 2018.
3. Australian Bureau of Statistics. *Causes of Death, Australia, 2019*; Australian Bureau of Statistics: Canberra, Australia, 2019.
4. Centre for Disease Control. *Excess Deaths Associated with COVID-19, 2020*; Centre for Disease Control: Atlanta, GA, USA, 2020.
5. Saar, E.; Bugeja, L.; Ranson, D.L. National Coronial Information System: Epidemiology and the Coroner in Australia. *Acad. Forensic Pathol.* **2017**, *7*, 582–590. [CrossRef] [PubMed]
6. Mikkelsen, L.; Iburg, K.M.; Adair, T.; Fürst, T.; Hegnauer, M.; von der Lippe, E.; Moran, L.; Nomura, S.; Sakamoto, H.; Shibuya, K.; et al. Assessing the quality of cause of death data in six high-income countries: Australia, Canada, Denmark, Germany, Japan and Switzerland. *Int. J. Public Health* **2020**, *65*, 17–28. [CrossRef] [PubMed]

7. Australian Bureau of Statistics. *Classifying Place of Death in Australian Mortality Statistics, 2021*; Australian Bureau of Statistics: Canberra, Australia, 2021.
8. Australian Bureau of Statistics. *Psychosocial Risk Factors as They Relate to Coroner-Referred Deaths in Australia, 2017*; Australian Bureau of Statistics: Canberra, Australia, 2017.
9. Australian Bureau of Statistics. *Provisional Mortality Statistics, January 2020–July 2021*; Australian Bureau of Statistics: Canberra, Australia, 2021.
10. Australian Bureau of Statistics. *Measuring Excess Mortality in Australia During the COVID-19 Pandemic*; Australian Bureau of Statistics: Canberra, Australia, 2020.
11. Islam, N.; Shkolnikov, V.M.; Acosta, R.J.; Klimkin, I.; Kawachi, I.; Irizarry, R.A.; Alicandro, G.; Khunti, K.; Yates, T.; Jdanov, D.A.; et al. Excess deaths associated with COVID-19 pandemic in 2020: Age and sex disaggregated time series analysis in 29 high income countries. *BMJ* **2021**, *373*, n1137. [CrossRef] [PubMed]
12. Matthew, K.; Gloria, M.; Chalapati, R. Lessons Learnt and Pathways forward for National Civil Registration and Vital Statistics Systems after the COVID-19 Pandemic. *J. Epidemiol. Glob. Health* **2021**, *11*, 262. [CrossRef]
13. World Health Organization. *ICD-11 Implementation or Transition Guide, 2019*; WHO: Geneva, Switzerland, 2019.
14. Federal Institute for Drugs and Medical Devices (BfArM). *ICD-11 Lessons from COVID-19, 2020*; Iris Institute: Cologne, Germany, 2020.

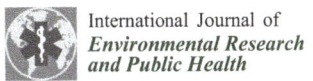

Review

Health and Access to Health Services for People with Disability in Australia: Data and Data Gaps

Nicola Fortune [1,2,*], Rosamond H. Madden [1] and Shane Clifton [1]

1. Centre for Disability Research and Policy, The University of Sydney, Susan Wakil Health Building, Western Ave., Camperdown, NSW 2050, Australia; ros.madden@sydney.edu.au (R.H.M.); drshaneclifton@gmail.com (S.C.)
2. Centre of Research Excellence in Disability and Health, University of Melbourne, 207 Bouverie Str., Carlton, VIC 3053, Australia
* Correspondence: nicola.fortune@sydney.edu.au

Abstract: The right of people with disability to enjoyment of the highest attainable standard of health without discrimination on the basis of disability is enshrined in the United Nations Convention on the Rights of Persons with Disabilities (CRPD). Among its obligations as a signatory to the CRPD, Australia is required to collect appropriate information, including statistical and research data, to inform development and implementation of policies to give effect to the Convention. In this commentary, we first describe how the International Classification of Functioning, Disability and Health (ICF) conceptual model of disability can be operationalised in statistical data collections, with a focus on how this is achieved in key Australian data sources such that people with disability can be identified as a population group. We then review existing statistical data on health and health service use for people with disability in Australia, highlighting data gaps and limitations. Finally, we outline priorities and considerations for improving data on health and access to health services for people with disability. As well as conceptual, practical, and ethical considerations, a key principle that must guide future disability data development is that people with disability and their representative organisations must be involved and participate fully in the development of disability data and statistics, and in their use.

Keywords: health services; disability; data gaps; disability identification; International Classification of Functioning, Disability and Health (ICF); Convention on the Rights of Persons with Disabilities (CRPD); health statistics; disability statistics; inequalities

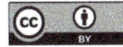

1. Introduction

People with disability have the right to enjoy the highest attainable standard of health without discrimination on the basis of disability, as affirmed in Article 25 of the United Nations Convention on the Rights of Persons with Disabilities (CRPD) [1]. This right is not currently being realised. In Australia, as in other countries across the globe, people with disability experience poorer health outcomes than people without disability [2–6]. At population level, disability-related health disparities are caused in large part by avoidable disadvantage, and not primarily by underlying impairment [7]. As such, governments have a duty to act to reduce these health disparities.

Population statistical data have a crucial role to play in identifying and understanding disability-related inequalities, informing more effective policy interventions, evaluating interventions, and holding key actors to account. Numerous international and Australian reports have highlighted the need for population-level statistical data that can be disaggregated by disability, and the importance of using such data for monitoring and regularly reporting on disability-related inequalities [6,8–10]. In Australia, the current policy context has generated a high level of interest in disability data. Key features of this context include the National Disability Insurance Scheme (which reached full rollout in July 2020), the ongoing Royal Commission into Violence, Abuse, Neglect and Exploitation of People with Disability, and the development of a new national disability strategy to guide Australian disability policy for the coming decade.

In the context of health systems and health data, disability has traditionally been treated as an outcome [11]. This is powerfully illustrated by the Global Burden of Disease study: an international epidemiological study that produces estimates of the fatal and non-fatal 'burden' attributable to specific diseases and risk factors using the Disability Adjusted Life Year (DALY) metric [12,13]. Considering health inequalities experienced by people with disability requires a wholly different perspective. It means viewing disability as akin to a demographic factor by which health data may be disaggregated [11]. However, the concept of disability is inextricably linked to and defined with reference to health. Thus, use of statistical data to investigate disability-related health inequalities presents complexities that require interrogation.

Statistical classifications provide standard structures for collecting, organising and analysing data [14]. The use of standard statistical classifications as a basis for developing data collections promotes data consistency, so that data from different sources may be compared and potentially used together to generate new information and boost the value of existing data resources. The World Health Organization's (WHO) Family of International Classifications is a suite of classifications designed to provide internationally consistent information on different aspects of health and the healthcare system [15]. The three core members of the WHO-FIC are the International Classification of Diseases (ICD), the International Classification of Functioning, Disability and Health (ICF), and the International Classification of Health Interventions (ICHI) (currently in development). The ICF has been broadly adopted as the international standard framework and classification for organising and documenting information about functioning and disability [16], and has been used in Australia to underpin the development of disability-related data items in population surveys and administrative data collections [17].

In this paper, we describe how people with disability are identified in key Australian data sources, review available statistical data on health and health service use for people with disability, and outline priorities and considerations to guide efforts to fill data gaps and improve the evidence base.

2. Methods

To inform this commentary, we searched for publications relevant to disability data on the websites of Australia's two main national statistics institutions—the Australian Bureau of Statistics and the Australian Institute of Health and Welfare. Reports and technical documents available from these websites provide information about data relevant to disability available in key statistical data sources, including detailed descriptions of how disability is operationally defined.

We also referred to an Audit of Disability Research in Australia, first conducted in 2014 and updated in 2017 [18]. Finally, we conducted a simple search on 'national disability statistics in Australia'. Our aim was to identify sources of statistical data in Australia relevant to health and health service use for people with disability, and related research.

3. Functioning, Disability and Health

The ICF was endorsed by all WHO Member States in the Fifty-fourth World Health Assembly in 2001. Its development was preceded and informed by decades of worldwide discussion involving a range of service providers, health professionals, and researchers, as well as people with disability and their representative organisations [19,20]. One of the main threads of these discussions was the recognition that the environment plays a significant role in the experience of disability.

The ICF defines the main components of functioning as body functions and structures, activities and participation. It provides classifications of body functions, body structures, activity and participation domains and environmental factors (see Box 1). Environmental factors have a crucial effect (as facilitators or barriers) on people's functioning and on the creation of disability in many life areas. The ICF represents a biopsychosocial model of disability, combining the medical and social models of disability, thus recognising that disability may require both treatment at the individual level, as well as social and environmental change [19,21]. It shows us a dynamic interaction between a person's health conditions and contextual factors—relationships that are probabilistic and not deterministic or linearly causal.

Box 1. Definitions of the components of the ICF, and of functioning and disability.

> **Body functions**—The physiological functions of body systems (including psychological functions). **Body structures**—Anatomical parts of the body, such as organs, limbs and their components. **Impairments**—Problems in body function or structure, such as a significant deviation or loss. **Activity**—The execution of a task or action by an individual. **Participation**—Involvement in a life situation. **Activity limitations**—Difficulties an individual may have in executing activities. **Participation restrictions**—Problems an individual may experience in involvement in life situations. **Environmental factors** make up the physical, social and attitudinal environment in which people live and conduct their lives. These are either barriers to or facilitators of the person's functioning. **Functioning** is an umbrella term encompassing all body functions, activities and participation. It denotes the positive or neutral aspects of the interaction between a person's health condition(s) and that individual's contextual factors (environmental and personal factors). **Disability** is an umbrella term for impairments, activity limitations and participation restrictions. It denotes the negative aspects of the interaction between a person's health condition(s) and that individual's contextual factors (environmental and personal factors). Source: WHO, 2001, pp. 3, 8, 10

The ICF was developed in the same era as the CRPD, with the former concerned with classification and data, and the latter with provision of human rights. The ICF and CRPD share common concepts, culture and terms (e.g., environment, barriers, participation), and the subject matter of rights in the CRPD can readily be mapped (or cross-walked) to the ICF domains, demonstrating that the two instruments have broad commonality of content [22,23]. The CRPD requires governments that have ratified the Convention to report on progress with achieving its aims—rights, access and equity—and to collect statistics to help formulate and implement policy and to monitor the Convention (*Articles 31, 33 and 35*). The ICF is designed to enable the collection and comparison of data relating to functioning and disability in many fields and across the world, and it provides a suitable framework to underpin monitoring the implementation of the CRPD [23,24].

Statistical classifications provide the building blocks for sound health information systems [25,26]. Over the past 20 years, the ICF has influenced functioning and disability information, measurement and statistics [24]. It is used in diverse applications, settings and countries. Nevertheless, it is considered that there is a need for "more applications of the full ICF model, including those that incorporate Environmental Factors into applications, such as surveys and measurement instruments" ([24], p.1455). The benefits of doing this are well illustrated by the first National Disability Survey in Ireland in 2006, with survey results showing the substantial impact of environmental factors on people's functioning [27]. The WHO has called for the wider use of the ICF to increase worldwide disability data quality and consistency [21,28,29].

Australia recognises both the moral and legal framework of the CRPD and the technical framework of the ICF. In 2008, Australia ratified the CRPD, and now makes links to CRPD objectives in major public policies and programs, such as the National Disability Strategy 2010–2020 and National Disability Insurance Scheme [30,31]. Any success of these initiatives should be indicated by relative improvements in participation by people with disability in many life areas and in access to services. The challenge for national statistics in any country is to produce reliable data capable of telling the story of participation, access and equity. Australian statistical organisations such as the ABS and the AIHW adhere to international standards to produce data that enable national and international comparisons, and to capture consistent administrative data nationally. Both organisations, before and since the publication of the ICF, have been advised on statistics and data standards by broadly-based groups that include disability advocacy organisations.

Measuring progress in fulfilling CRPD goals requires data that can be used to compare the experiences of people with disability with those of people without disability, for example, in employment, housing, or access to health services. The ICF does not divide people dichotomously into 'disabled' and 'not disabled'. Therefore, methods are required that enable population data to be disaggregated into groups, according to people's level of functioning. Such methods should be designed to suit the purpose and context, for example, to define eligibility for services, to estimate disability prevalence, or to monitor progress towards achieving equity.

How can the ICF conception of disability as a dynamic interaction between a person's health conditions and contextual factors (personal and environmental) be best operationalised in statistical data collections, to enable the production of data for people 'with' and 'without' disability? The first step is to identify the main questions of interest—those that lend themselves to measurement and quantification—and to articulate the main related purposes and methods to be used [32]. Statistical design and analysis can then draw on the clarity and simplification offered by the classifications of the ICF to help frame the concepts underlying the questions on which evidence is sought and specify relevant data items.

Defining 'disability status' is not straightforward, given that:

"The ICF puts the notions of 'health' and 'disability' in a new light. It acknowledges that every human being can experience some disability. ... ICF thus 'mainstreams' the experience of disability and recognizes it as a universal human experience. By shifting the focus from cause to impact, it places all health conditions on an equal footing, allowing them to be compared using a common metric—the ruler of health and disability." ([27], p. 1068)

Designing an operational definition of disability is a complex task that is sometimes implied or simplified rather than fully explicated. A description of the method used in the World Report on Disability illustrates some key points in a general methodology [16]. The method entailed creating a spectrum of difficulty with activities and designing 'cut points' in a transparent way, to indicate what is included in the definition of 'disability' used for estimation purposes ([27], p. 1066). Similarly, the Model Disability Survey was developed by WHO to collect 'comprehensive, comparable and relevant disability information' to monitor the CRPD. It aims to capture 'how people actually function in multiple domains, given the environmental barriers and facilitators that constitute their real life situation', by asking about 'problems in daily life' ([33], pp.4-5). The data are used to generate a continuum ranging from low to high levels of disability—a metrical scale developed using Item Response Theory. This disability distribution can be partitioned using cut-points to define groups with no, mild, moderate and severe disability for data disaggregation purposes.

Since it was first run in 1982, the Australian Survey of Disability Ageing and Carers (SDAC) has been used to provide prevalence estimates of disability and profiles of people (including older people) who experience difficulties functioning in everyday life. SDAC follows the ICF framework and, broadly speaking, its definitions. Inclusion into the survey is via screening questions focused on a list of long-term health conditions, impairments and activity limitations, including 'any other health conditions resulting in a restriction'. Survey respondents are then asked an array of questions, including about difficulty with everyday activities [34,35]. The Survey publications present data on disability in terms of the difficulties people experience in areas of daily life, as well as their impairments and long-term health conditions. The main environmental factor which informs SDAC's definitions of disability is 'assistance'. The Survey's concepts of severe or profound core activity limitation relate to a person's need for assistance with 'core activities', namely self-care, mobility and communication [35]. The operational definition of disability in SDAC is 'any limitation, restriction or impairment which restricts everyday activities and has lasted, or is likely to last, for at least six months' [36].

The SDAC methodology thus accords with that recommended by WHO authors and colleagues ([27], p. 1068): " ... disability surveys should rely on a broad range of questions covering the whole range of the experience of functioning—bodily impairments, activity limitations, participation restrictions and environmental facilitators or barriers. Arguably, the final intention of health and health related interventions is to maximize functioning in a person's lived environment and hence disability surveys are best focused on measuring the person's functioning in interaction with his or her environment".

Several other ABS social surveys include a 'Short Disability Module' of 16 questions that aims to identify people with disability and their limitations and restrictions in a way that aligns with SDAC [34]. A 'Core Activity Need for Assistance' module has been included in the Australian Census since 2006, to measure the number of people 'needing help or assistance in one or more of the three core activity areas of self-care, mobility and communication, because of a long-term health condition (lasting six months or more), a disability (lasting six months or more), or old age' [37]. It is designed to align conceptually with severe or profound core activity limitation in SDAC.

The use of common concepts and data standards relating to disability across population surveys and administrative data collections provides a basis for relating data from different sources. Australia's disability services national minimum dataset, established in the early 2000s, included a 'support needs' data item based on the ICF activities and participation domains and the SDAC question on need for personal help or supervision with activities or participation in particular life areas [38]. The resulting data from the national disability services data collection could be related to SDAC data, which enabled some powerful analyses bringing together data on users of disability services with SDAC data on the target population to produce estimates and projections of met and unmet need for support [39]. Provision of disability services in Australia has now transitioned to the National Disability Insurance Scheme. Legislation governing eligibility for the Scheme requires that assessment tools used must "have reference to areas of activity and social and economic participation identified in the World Health Organisation International Classification of Functions, Disability and Health" ([40], 7.5(b)).

SDAC data are accessible to researchers external to the ABS, thus enabling wider use of the data. Data have been used, for example, to illuminate rights-related issues, such as the experience of disability discrimination, prevalence of disability among Indigenous Australians, and access to services by Australians of diverse cultures [41–43].

The CRPD sets out the rights of people with disability to access all services available to society as a whole. Creating a succinct disability 'identifier' for use in administrative data collections is a key challenge for public policy design and monitoring in any country [16,23,44]. Meeting this challenge involves the design and adoption of short question sets, ideally a single question, to identify people with disability consistently within service data systems, so that it is possible to monitor equity of access, participation and outcomes [45,46].

4. Data on Health and Health Service Use for People with Disability

According to SDAC 2018 data, more than 4 million Australians have disability, or around 18% of the population [2]. Lack of equitable and timely access to appropriate health care, especially preventive care and proactive management of health risks and chronic conditions, has been identified as a factor contributing to poor health outcomes for people with disability [4]. Submissions to Australia's Royal Commission into Violence, Abuse, Neglect and Exploitation of People with Disability highlight barriers to equitable and timely access to quality health care for people with disability, particularly for those with cognitive disability and Aboriginal and Torres Strait Islander people with disability [47–51]. Barriers cited include inadequate staff training, expertise and capacity, limited access to skilled patient advocates, costs, accessibility of buildings and health care equipment (e.g., mammography machines), and discriminatory attitudes. There has long been recognition of the need to address health inequalities, and barriers to accessing appropriate health services, particularly for people with intellectual disability [52].

For people with disability, as for all people, health is a key enabler of participation across all domains of life, and health services, systems and policies are environmental factors that can play a critical role as facilitators of or barriers to participation. The Australian Health Performance Framework (AHPF) is used to assess the health of Australia's population and performance of the health system [53–55]. It has four broad domains—Health status, Determinants of health, Health system, and Health system context. The principle of equity overarches these domains. To determine whether equity is being achieved, statistical data are required that enable indicators to be reported for particular population sub-groups, including people with disability.

4.1. What Do We Know about Health Conditions Experienced by People with Disability?

National population surveys provide data on health conditions experienced by people with and without disability. In SDAC, the survey modules used for disability identification ask respondents what is the main condition that causes each of the impairments or activity limitations they report. Respondents are then asked if they are receiving treatment for any long-term condition and whether they have any other long-term condition. Due to the structure of the survey questions in SDAC, there is an emphasis on health conditions that are associated with impairments and limitations. SDAC data have been used to report on rates of disability associated with particular health conditions, and on associations between health conditions and particular limitations and impairments [2,56–58]. For example, for people aged under 65 years in 2003, the health conditions with the highest associated rates of profound or severe core activity limitations were autism (82%), paralysis (79%), and speech-related conditions (67%); for people aged under 65 with severe or profound core activity limitations, the most common health conditions were back problems and arthritis, consistent with their high prevalence in the general population ([58], pp. 223–225).

The ABS National Health Survey also provides data on long-term health conditions, and identifies people with disability using the ABS short disability module. Table 1 presents data from the 2017–2018 National Health Survey for the 20 most common groups of current, long-term health conditions reported by all people aged 15–64 years, and compares prevalence for people with and without disability. 'Disorders of ocular muscles, binocular movement accommodation & refraction' were most prevalent, with similar rates for people with and without disability (65% and 62%, respectively). For all other condition groups listed, rates were higher for people with disability than for those without disability. For 11 condition groups, the rate for people with disability was more than twice that for people without disability. The rate for people with disability was more than three times that for people without disability for anxiety related problems, mood disorders, partial deafness and hearing loss, and other diseases of the ear.

National Health Survey data also reveal higher rates of multi-morbidity for people with disability compared to people without disability in 2017–2018. For people aged 15–24 years, the median number of current, long-term conditions reported was three for those with disability, compared to one for those without; for people aged 25–64 years, the median number of conditions was four for those with disability, compared to one for those without; and for people in the age groups 50–64 years and 65 years and over, the median number of conditions was six for those with disability, compared to three for those without.

These differences between people with and without disability in rates of long-term health conditions and multi-morbidity are not unexpected, given the relationship between health conditions and disability, discussed above. However, such data can shed light on the potential health-related needs of people with disability compared to those without disability. More detailed insights can be gained by breaking down the data, for example, by gender, disability group, disability severity, or area of residence (urban/non-urban). Such information is relevant for guiding health policy. For example, considering the higher rates of diabetes among people with disability, together with the prevalence of disability in the population, it is clear that diabetes prevention or management interventions must be accessible and appropriate for people with disability, otherwise they will not be effective for a substantial portion of the target population [11].

These data do not, however, provide insights into the extent to which higher rates of some conditions may be related to the right of equal access to healthcare not being met for people with disability, for instance, because of barriers to accessing primary and secondary prevention.

Table 1. Prevalence of the 20 most commonly reported [1] current, long-term health conditions, by disability status, for people aged 15–64 years (National Health Survey 2017–2018).

Health Condition Group	Disability (95% CI)	No Disability [2] (95% CI)	Rate Ratio [3] (95% CI)
1. Disorders of ocular muscles binocular movement accommodation & refraction	65% (63, 67)	62% (61, 63)	1.0 (1.0, 1.1)
2. Other diseases of respiratory system	32% (30, 34)	25% (24, 26)	1.3 (1.2, 1.4)
3. Dorsopathies	37% (35, 39)	13% (12, 14)	2.9 (2.6, 3.2)
4. Symptoms, signs and conditions not elsewhere classified (NEC)	24% (22, 25)	12% (11, 13)	1.9 (1.8, 2.1)
5. Anxiety related problems	29% (27, 31)	9% (8, 10)	3.4 (3.0, 3.8)
6. Mood (affective) disorders	29% (27, 31)	7% (6, 8)	4.2 (3.6, 4.8)
7. Arthropathies	28% (26, 29)	10% (9, 11)	2.7 (2.5, 3.0)
8. Chronic lower respiratory diseases	20% (18, 22)	9% (9, 10)	2.1 (1.8, 2.4)
9. Episodic & paroxysmal disorders	18% (16, 19)	6% (5, 7)	3.0 (2.6, 3.4)
10. Hypertensive disease	13% (12, 15)	8% (7, 9)	1.6 (1.4, 1.8)
11. Partial deafness & hearing loss (NEC)	20% (19, 21)	3% (3, 4)	5.7 (4.7, 6.6)
12. Other endocrine, nutritional & metabolic diseases	10% (9, 12)	5% (5, 6)	2.0 (1.6, 2.3)
13. Other diseases of the ear	10% (9, 12)	2% (2, 3)	4.1 (3.1, 5.1)
14. Diseases of the skin and subcutaneous tissue	6% (5, 7)	4% (3, 4)	1.6 (1.2, 2.0)
15. Diabetes mellitus	6% (5, 7)	4% (3, 4)	1.7 (1.4, 2.1)
16. Disorders of thyroid gland	6% (5, 7)	4% (3, 4)	1.6 (1.2, 1.9)
17. Diseases of genito-urinary system	6% (5, 7)	3% (2, 3)	2.3 (1.7, 2.8)
18. Other diseases of eye & adnexa	4% (3, 5)	3% (2, 3)	1.4 (1.1, 1.8)
19. Diseases of the oesophagus, stomach & duodenum	5% (4, 6)	2% (1, 2)	2.6 (1.9, 3.3)
20. Diseases of blood and blood forming organs	4% (3, 4)	2% (1, 2)	2.1 (1.6, 2.7)

[1] Based on health conditions reported by all people aged 15–64 years. [2] Prevalence rates for people with 'no disability' are age-standardised to the age structure of the population with disability; these rates should be interpreted as the hypothetical rates that would have been observed if the population without disability had the same age structure as the population with disability. [3] Rate ratio is calculated as: (% for people with disability)/(% for people without disability). Source: Australian Bureau of Statistics (2019) Microdata: National Health Survey, 2017–2018 (DataLab), accessed July 2021.

4.2. What Do We Know about Contact with Health Services by People with Disability?

Population surveys capture some information on contact with health services by people with disability. For instance, the National Health Survey (2017–18) provides data on the proportion of people who consulted different types of health professionals in the past 12 months. Compared to people without disability aged 18–64 years, a higher percentage of those with disability reported having consulted a GP (92%, compared with 83% of those without disability), a specialist (50%, compared with 29% of those without disability), and an allied health professional (37%, compared with 19% of those without disability) [59]. In the 2014 General Social Survey, a higher proportion of people with disability reported experiencing a barrier to accessing healthcare when needed (15%), compared to those without disability (3%); the proportion was higher still for people with severe or profound core activity limitation (24%) [59]. SDAC provides data on the proportion of people with disability who report unmet need for different types of health services, and who report cost as a barrier to accessing health services [2]; but these data are not collected for people without disability, so comparison is not possible.

While valuable, survey data on contact with health services, barriers, and unmet needs have a number of limitations. First, the available information is based on quite broad questions, so tends to lack specificity. Second, surveys capture a snapshot at certain points in time (e.g., every 3 years in the case of SDAC). Thirdly, the ability to conduct analyses focusing on particular subgroups of people with disability may be limited due to small sample size. Fourthly, the reliability of the information is dependent on the accuracy of respondents' memory and perceptions about their interactions with health services.

In addition, survey sample frames for many ABS surveys do not cover people living in Very Remote Areas, in discrete Aboriginal and Torres Strait Islander communities, or in non-private dwellings. The ABS list of non-private dwellings includes boarding houses, hospitals, psychiatric hospitals or institutions, hostels for the disabled, nursing homes, accommodation for people who are homeless, prisons, and other welfare institutions (including group homes for people with disability) [37,60]. SDAC provides limited data on people who live in health establishments that provide long-term cared accommodation, but the questionnaire used for this survey component focuses on health conditions, core activities, use of aids, and assistance provided, and is completed by a staff member for each selected occupant; the data do not cover broader topics relating to contact with health services, participation across life domains, or social and economic outcomes.

Administrative data sources are an important complement to survey data for population heath research, as they can provide more detailed and comprehensive data on service users. Currently, in Australia, no national health services administrative datasets include disability identification. Therefore, it is not possible to produce policy-relevant data on contact with health services for people with disability and associated outcomes, or to make comparisons between people with and without disability to determine whether the AHPF objective of equity is being attained.

The National Hospitals Data Collection includes a number of databases that contain episode-level information on hospital care provided to admitted and non-admitted patients (https://www.aihw.gov.au/about-our-data/our-data-collections/national-hospitals; accessed on 5 November 2021). These databases are used for reporting on AHPF indicators, including rates of hospitalisation for injury and poisoning, hospitalisations involving an adverse event, selected potentially preventable hospitalisations, in-hospital falls, hospitalisation rates for selected procedures, waiting time to admission for selected elective surgery procedures, and emergency department presentations seen on time. None of these measures can be broken down by disability status, as there is no disability identifier in these data sources.

Consistent national data on primary health care (including GP visits) is currently not available. Data captured in patient electronic health records are not currently suitable for conducting reliable or representative analyses at regional, state or national levels, due to data quality, comparability and access issues [61,62]. Data from the now discontinued Bettering the Evaluation and Care of Health (BEACH) collection have been used to examine GP encounters for patients with intellectual disability and autism spectrum disorder, with analyses indicating that these patient groups differed from other patients in terms of demographic characteristics, reasons for encounter, consultation type, consultation length, problems managed, medications, treatments provided, and referrals made [63–65].

The Department of Health publishes statistics on services provided under Australia's Medicare scheme (available to all Australians), for example, bulk-billing rates, average patient contributions, and broad service types (e.g., optometry, other allied health, diagnostic imaging). However, Medicare data cannot be broken down by patient disability status. (https://www1.health.gov.au/internet/main/publishing.nsf/Content/Medicare%20Statistics-1; accessed on 5 November 2021).

4.3. The Future Potential of Linked Administrative Data

Linked administrative datasets offer potential for filling some data gaps. The principle is that individual-level disability-identifying information captured in one dataset is linked with individual-level records in other datasets to enable analyses focusing on people with disability. This approach has been used in two Australian states to examine service use and related outcomes for people with intellectual disability [66–70], and to analyse mortality data for people with autism spectrum disorders [71]. For example, use of linked data to examine health service use in the last year of life for a matched cohort of people with and without intellectual disability in Western Australia found that people with intellectual disability attended emergency departments more frequently, were admitted to hospital less frequently, had longer hospital stays, and had increased odds of presentation, admission or death associated with potentially preventable conditions [72]. Similarly, a large New South Wales cohort study using linked data found intellectual disability to be associated with higher rates of emergency department presentations, psychiatric readmissions, premature mortality, and potentially avoidable deaths, and with longer length of stay in psychiatric units [66].

While data linkage has an important role to play in improving the evidence base, it must be understood that identification of people with disability in linked datasets will be limited by disability identifying information available in the constituent datasets. This is likely often to include identification based on receipt of disability-related services or income support payments. The majority of people with disability do not receive disability-related services or payments [2]. Thus, without a means of identifying people with disability more comprehensively in administrative data, information on equity of access to health and other services will remain incomplete.

5. Moving Forward: Some Key Considerations

We have outlined how the ICF model of disability is operationalised in data collections in Australia, to enable the disaggregation of population data by disability status, and we have provided an overview of available data on health and health service use for people with disability. It is clear that work is needed to address existing data gaps and limitations, to more fully understand the experiences of people with disability in relation to health and health services, to measure disability-related inequalities, and to monitor implementation of Article 25 of the CRPD. In this section, we raise some key considerations that must be kept front-of-mind as Australia moves forward with data development in this area.

There is a long history of research labelling, pathologising, and dehumanising people with disability [73,74]. The collection and use of statistical data is not a neutral exercise [75]. Just as the indigenous data sovereignty movement is a response to the statistical narrative of deficit and dysfunction that has framed the portrayal of indigenous peoples globally [76], so too are people with disability looking to take leadership over the way disability research is conducted, reported and utilised. Emerging out of the disability rights movement of the 1970s and 1980s, the discipline of disability studies builds on the logic of "nothing about us without us" to insist that only the active involvement of people with disability can protect research from the paternalism and medicalisation that has plagued its history. Co-produced research (often called inclusive research in the context of intellectual disability [77,78]) looks to guard against ableist bias and ensure that research is focused on social systems rather than individual deficits [79].

While the ICF itself is a product of the emerging disability rights movement, diligence is needed to ensure it is not used to label, classify and control people with disability. The ethical guidelines for the use of the ICF require respect for the autonomy of people with disability and their involvement in the collection and use of data ([21], Annex 6). These ideas can be deepened by including researchers with lived experience of disability and partnering with Disabled People's Organisations in research design and the development of disability data and statistics, and in the use of data for informing public policy.

Among the ethical considerations that should guide the collection and reporting of statistical data on health and access to health services for people with disability is the need to ensure all cohorts of people are captured in data that will shape public policy. This requirement can be in tension with decisions to be made about research participation, such as the need to prevent coercion and judge the capacity for consent [80–82]. Contrary to common ableist presumptions (including among ethics committees) [83,84], it should be assumed that people with disability are capable of providing consent unless established otherwise [80]. Those gathering data have the responsibility to promote understanding about the purpose and intended use of the data ([21], Annex 6). This may require implementing supported decision-making practices, and tailoring approaches for gathering data that utilise mechanisms to facilitate understanding such as Easy Read [85,86].

Notwithstanding capacity to consent, many people with disability are reliant on gatekeepers, such as parents, support workers, and institutional managers, who may prevent or constrain their interaction with people gathering data [87]. Gatekeepers may be concerned about the impact of research upon 'vulnerable' people, and suspicious of its benefits. While suspicion of research and data collection is not without reason, overemphasis on protection discounts the harm of paternalism and undermines the rights of people with disability to participate in research that can inform improved disability policy and practices [86]. Both gatekeepers and people with disability themselves may be concerned that the information they provide could affect the way they are treated and their eligibility for supports [86]. As stated in the ICF ethical guidelines, data collected should enhance choices and control, support, and participation of people in the community, and not be employed to restrict people's rights or entitlements ([21], Annex 6). Likewise, Article 31 of the CRPD requires the collection and use of statistical data to give effect to the rights set out in the Convention.

While confidentiality and privacy are central principles in the collection and management of data about individuals, some people with disability rely upon and trust their support workers, and depend upon their help in participating in research and providing data. Successful data collection is thus dependent upon fostering trust among complex stakeholder networks, utilising support to conduct research while collecting data using strict safeguards for identification, storage, and publication that protect participants from any negative consequences [80,86].

The challenges of collecting health data from and about people with disability are magnified in segregated institutional settings under the control of gatekeepers, yet monitoring of health is especially important in such settings. Particular mention should be made here of the criminal justice system. People with disability are known to be over-represented in the criminal justice system, with consequent negative health impacts [66,88–90], especially for those exposed to intersectional discrimination such as Aboriginal and Torres Strait Islander people with disability [91]. There is also evidence that justice systems often fail to identify offenders with intellectual disability [89,90]. Thus, to ensure rights to health and health services are upheld, strategies are needed to ensure the full representation of people with disability within these settings.

Producing statistics is not just a technical endeavour. We have already identified the centrality of co-producing health data with people with disability, and this rationale extends to including the insight of people with disability and other intersectional health disadvantages, such as racial, sexual, gendered, and aged. For example, Aboriginal and Torres Strait Islander people with disability experience multilayered disadvantage from racism and ableism, and collecting and publishing health statistics on this cohort of people is thus vital and complex [92]. It involves recognition of cultural, social, political and ethical dimensions of research with First Peoples with disability, especially their right to self-determination, and culturally safe and inclusive research practices [93,94].

6. Conclusions

In Australia, we are fortunate to have established population data sources with disability identifiers that are conceptually aligned with the ICF. This is a result of sustained resourcing by government, the work of statistical agencies (particularly ABS and AIHW), and active input from people with disability and other stakeholders. Nonetheless, important data gaps and limitations remain, hampering Australia's ability to develop effective policy responses to uphold the rights of people with disability, especially in relation to health and access to health services.

Moving forward to address these data gaps and limitations, the challenge is to develop an array of sources, with relatable data on disability. Clear articulation of the purpose for which data are to be used is crucial to guide any data development work, but particularly in relation to identifying people with disability, and deciding where and how to place 'cut points' along the continuum of functioning to define different groups. The corollary of this is that the purpose for which a particular data source has been designed must be understood and taken into account when considering secondary use of the data, including in the context of data linkage.

Disability data development should adhere to well-established principles, such as using data standards to promote quality and consistency, the importance of consultation, collaboration and field testing, being aware of the limitations of the data, and weighing the costs of data collection to all concerned against the value gained [17,95,96].

Building an effective evidence base to inform better policy and practice requires that data from different sources are relatable and have sound conceptual underpinnings; ICF remains the relevant standard framework in relation to disability. However, developing data is never merely a technical endeavour: there must always be consideration of the cultural, social, political and ethical dimensions, and the implications for those to whom the data relate. Crucially, people with disability and their representative organisations must be key players in the development of disability data and statistics, and in their use.

Finally, good data rely on ongoing, active input from all parties who have an interest in the data. We encourage disability advocates, researchers, and policy makers to use the valuable disability data sources available in Australia, with an awareness of the concepts underpinning these data, and to engage in ongoing discussions and efforts to improve our national disability data resources into the future.

Author Contributions: Conceptualization, N.F. and R.H.M.; investigation, N.F., R.H.M. and S.C.; writing—original draft, N.F., R.H.M. and S.C.; writing—review and editing, N.F., R.H.M. and S.C. All authors have read and agreed to the published version of the manuscript.

Funding: This research received no external funding.

Institutional Review Board Statement: Not applicable.

Informed Consent Statement: Not applicable.

Data Availability Statement: ABS survey data cited in this paper are available to researchers for analysis, see https://www.abs.gov.au/websitedbs/d3310114.nsf/home/microdata+entry+page (accessed on 5 November 2021).

Conflicts of Interest: The authors declare no conflict of interest.

References

1. United Nations. Convention on the Rights of Persons with Disabilities. Available online: www.un.org/development/desa/disabilities/convention-on-the-rights-of-persons-with-disabilities.html (accessed on 5 November 2021).
2. Australian Institute of Health and Welfare. *People with Disability in Australia 2020*; AIHW: Canberra, Australia, 2020.
3. Australian Institute of Health and Welfare. *Mortality Patterns Among People Using Disability Support Services: 1 July 2013 to 30 June 2018*; Technical Report. Cat. No. DIS 76; AIHW: Canberra, Australia, 2020.

4. Salomon, C.; Trollor, J. *A Scoping Review of Causes and Contributors to Deaths of People with Disability in Australia (2013–2019). Exhibit 4-059-CTD.7200.0001.0060 3DN, UNSW. Report for the Royal Commission into Violence, Abuse, Neglect and Exploitation of People with Disability*; University of New South Wales: Sydney, Australia, 2019.
5. Trollor, J.; Small, J. *Health Inequality and People with Intellectual Disability—Research Summary*; Faculty of Medicine, The Department of Developmental Disability Neuropsychiatry, UNSW: Sydney, Australia, 2019.
6. United Nations. *Disability and Development Report: Realizing the Sustainable Development Goals by, for and with Persons with Disabilities, 2018*; UN: New York, NY, USA, 2019.
7. Krahn, G.L.; Walker, D.K.; Correa-De-Araujo, R. Persons with disabilities as an unrecognized health disparity population. *Am. J. Public Health* **2015**, *105*, S198–S206. [CrossRef] [PubMed]
8. United Nations Committee on the Rights of Persons with Disabilities. *Concluding Observations on the Combined Second and Third Periodic Reports of Australia*; UN: New York, NY, USA, 2019.
9. Davy, L.; Fisher, K.; Wehbe, A.; Purcal, C.; Robinson, S.; Kayess, R.; Santos, D. *Review of Implementation of the National Disability Strategy 2010–2020. Final Report*; Social Policy Research Centre, UNSW: Sydney, Australia, 2018.
10. Civil Society CRPD Shadow Report Working Group. Disability Rights Now 2019. Australian Civil Society Shadow Report to the United Nations Committee on the Rights of Persons with Disabilities: UN CRPD Review 2019. Available online: https://pwd.org.au/our-work/policy-areas/human-rights-campaigns/united-nations-convention-on-the-rights-of-persons-with-disabilities/crpd-civil-society-shadow-report/ (accessed on 5 November 2021).
11. Krahn, G. Where is disability in global public health? In *Oxford Research Encyclopedia of Global Public Health*; Oxford University Press: Oxford, UK, 2021.
12. Moon, L.; Gourley, M.; Goss, J.; On, M.L.; Laws, P.; Reynolds, A.; Juckes, R. History and development of national burden of disease assessment in Australia. *Arch. Public Health* **2020**, *78*, 88. [CrossRef] [PubMed]
13. Vos, T.; Lim, S.S.; Abbafati, C.; Abbas, K.M.; Abbasi, M.; Abbasifard, M.; Abbasi-Kangevari, M.; Abbastabar, H.; Abd-Allah, F.; Abdelalim, A. Global burden of 369 diseases and injuries in 204 countries and territories, 1990–2019: A systematic analysis for the Global Burden of Disease Study 2019. *Lancet* **2020**, *396*, 1204–1222. [CrossRef]
14. Hancock, A. Best Practice Guidelines for Developing International Statistical Classifications. United Nations Department of Economic and Social Affairs Statistics Division. Expert Group Meeting on International Statistical Classifications. New York, 13–15 May 2013. Available online: https://unstats.un.org/unsd/classifications/bestpractices/Best_practice_Nov_2013.pdf (accessed on 5 November 2021).
15. World Health Organization. *International Statistical Classification of Diseases and Related Health Problems*, 5th ed.; 10th Revision, Instruction Manual; WHO: Geneva, Switzerland, 2016; Volume 2.
16. World Health Organization; World Bank. *World Report on Disability*; WHO: Geneva, Switzerland, 2011.
17. Madden, R.; Madden, R. Disability services and statistics: Past, present and future. In *Australia's Welfare 2019 Data Insights*; Australian Institute of Health and Welfare, Ed.; AIHW: Canberra, Australia, 2019.
18. Centre for Disability Research and Policy. *Audit of Disability Research in Australia Update Report 2017*; University of Sydney: Sydney, Australia, 2017.
19. Ustun, T.B.; Chatterji, S.; Bickenbach, J.; Kostanjsek, N.; Schneider, M. The International Classification of Functioning, Disability and Health: A new tool for understanding disability and health. *Disabil Rehabil* **2003**, *25*, 565–571. [CrossRef] [PubMed]
20. Schneidert, M.; Hurst, R.; Miller, J.; Üstün, B. The role of environment in the International Classification of Functioning, Disability and Health (ICF). *Disabil. Rehabil.* **2003**, *25*, 588–595. [CrossRef] [PubMed]
21. World Health Organization. *International Classification of Functioning, Disability and Health*; WHO: Geneva, Switzerland, 2001.
22. Bickenbach, J.E. Disability, culture and the UN convention. *Disabil. Rehabil.* **2009**, *31*, 1111–1124. [CrossRef] [PubMed]
23. Bickenbach, J.E. Monitoring the United Nation's Convention on the Rights of Persons with Disabilities: Data and the International Classification of Functioning, Disability and Health. *BMC Public Health* **2011**, *11* (Suppl. 4), S8. [CrossRef]
24. Madden, R.H.; Bundy, A. The ICF has made a difference to functioning and disability measurement and statistics. *Disabil. Rehabil.* **2018**, *41*, 1450–1462. [CrossRef]
25. United Nations. Fundamental Principles of Official Statistics (A/RES/68/261 from January 2014). Available online: https://unstats.un.org/fpos/ (accessed on 7 September 2021).
26. Madden, R.; Sykes, C.; Üstün, B. *World Health Organization Family of International Classifications: Definition, Scope and Purpose*; WHO: Geneva, Switzerland, 2007.
27. Kostanjsek, N.; Good, A.; Madden, R.H.; Üstün, T.B.; Chatterji, S.; Mathers, C.D.; Officer, A. Counting disability: Global and national estimation. *Disabil. Rehabil.* **2013**, *35*, 1065–1069. [CrossRef]
28. World Health Organization. How to Use the ICF: A Practical Manual for Using the International Classification of Functioning, Disability and Health (ICF). Exposure Draft for Comment. Available online: http://www.who.int/entity/classifications/drafticfpracticalmanual2.pdf?ua=1 (accessed on 7 September 2021).
29. World Health Organization. *WHO Global Disability Action Plan 2014–2021. Better Health for All People with Disability*; WHO: Geneva, Switzerland, 2015.
30. Commonwealth of Australia. *2010–2020 National Disability Strategy. An initiative of the Council of Australian Governments*; Commonwealth of Australia: Canberra, Australia, 2011.

31. National Disability Insurance Scheme Act 2013 (Cth). Available online: https://www.legislation.gov.au/Details/C2020C00392 (accessed on 7 September 2021).
32. Madden, R.; Fortune, N.; Cheeseman, D.; Mpofu, E.; Bundy, A. Fundamental questions before recording or measuring functioning and disability. *Disabil. Rehabil.* **2013**, *35*, 1092–1096. [CrossRef]
33. World Health Organization. *Model Disability Survey (MDS): Survey Manual*; Licence: CC BY-NC-SA 3.0 IGO; WHO: Geneva, Switzerland, 2017.
34. Australian Bureau of Statistics. *4431.0.55.002—ABS Sources of Disability Information, 2012–2016*; ABS: Canberra, Australia, 2018.
35. Australian Bureau of Statistics. *Disability, Ageing and Carers, Australia: Summary of Findings Methodology, 2018*; ABS: Canberra, Australia, 2019. Available online: https://www.abs.gov.au/methodologies/disability-ageing-and-carers-australia-summary-findings/2018 (accessed on 7 November 2021).
36. Australian Bureau of Statistics. *4430.0—Disability, Ageing and Carers, Australia: Summary of Findings, 2018*; ABS: Canberra, Australia, 2019. Available online: https://www.abs.gov.au/statistics/health/disability/disability-ageing-and-carers-australia-summary-findings/latest-release (accessed on 7 November 2021).
37. Australian Bureau of Statistics. *2901.0—Census of Population and Housing: Census Dictionary, 2016*; ABS: Canberra, Australia, 2016.
38. Anderson, P.; Madden, R. Design and quality of ICF-compatible data items for national disability support services. *Disabil. Rehabil.* **2011**, *33*, 758–769. [CrossRef]
39. Australian Institute of Health and Welfare. *Current and Future Demand for Specialist Disability Services*; Disability Series. Cat. No. DIS 50; AIHW: Canberra, Australia, 2007.
40. Australian Government. National Disability Insurance Scheme (Becoming a Participant) Rules. 2016. Available online: https://www.legislation.gov.au/Details/F2018C00165 (accessed on 5 November 2021).
41. Coleman, C.; Man, N.W.Y.; Gilroy, J.; Madden, R. Aboriginal and Torres Strait Islander disability prevalence: Making sense of multiple estimates and definitions. *Aust. N. Z. J. Public Health* **2018**, *42*, 562–566. [CrossRef]
42. Temple, J.B.; Kelaher, M.; Williams, R. Discrimination and avoidance due to disability in Australia: Evidence from a National Cross Sectional Survey. *BMC Public Health* **2018**, *18*, 1347. [CrossRef]
43. Zhou, Q. Accessing disability services by people from culturally and linguistically diverse backgrounds in Australia. *Disabil. Rehabil.* **2016**, *38*, 844–852. [CrossRef]
44. Verbrugge, L.M.; Jette, A.M. The disablement process. *Soc. Sci. Med.* **1994**, *38*, 1–14. [CrossRef]
45. Madden, R.; Choi, C.; Sykes, C. The ICF as a framework for national data: The introduction of ICF into Australian data dictionaries. *Disabil. Rehabil.* **2003**, *25*, 676–682. [CrossRef]
46. Madden, R.H.; Lukersmith, S.; Zhou, Q.; Glasgow, M.; Johnston, S. Disability-related questions for administrative datasets. *Int. J. Environ. Res. Public Health* **2020**, *17*, 5435. [CrossRef]
47. Lowitja Institute. Submission to the Royal Commission into Violence, Abuse, Neglect and Exploitation of People with Disability. Issues Paper: Health Care for People with Cognitive Disability. May 2020. Available online: https://disability.royalcommission.gov.au/publications/iss00100228 (accessed on 5 November 2021).
48. New South Wales Ageing and Disability Commission. Submission to the Royal Commission into Violence, Abuse, Neglect and Exploitation of People with Disability. Issues Paper: Health Care for People with Cognitive Disability. February 2020. Available online: https://disability.royalcommission.gov.au/publications/iss00100038 (accessed on 5 November 2021).
49. Royal Australian College of General Practitioners. RACGP Submission to the Royal Commission into Violence, Abuse, Neglect and Exploitation of People with Disability. Issues Paper: Healthcare for People with Cognitive Disability. April 2020. Available online: https://www.racgp.org.au/getmedia/06c7a743-30aa-42c5-b53b-6a4b629ab222/RACGP-submission-Healthcare-for-people-with-cognitive-disability.pdf.aspx (accessed on 5 November 2021).
50. Queensland Aboriginal and Islander Health Council. QAIHC Submission to the Royal Commission into Violence, Abuse, Neglect and Exploitation of People with Disability. April 2020. Available online: https://www.qaihc.com.au/media/37598/200406-submission-health-care-for-people-with-cognitive-disability-v11-final-20200407.pdf (accessed on 5 November 2021).
51. Avery, S. Royal Commission into Violence, Abuse, Neglect and Exploitation of People with Disability. Statement of Dr Scott Avery. 14 February 2020. Available online: https://disability.royalcommission.gov.au/publications/exhibit-4-18-stat006500010001-statement-dr-scott-avery (accessed on 7 November 2021).
52. Beange, H.; Lennox, N.; Parmenter, T.R. Health targets for people with an intellectual disability. *J. Intellect. Dev. Disabil.* **1999**, *24*, 283–297. [CrossRef]
53. Australian Institute of Health and Welfare. *Australia's Health 2018*; AIHW: Canberra, Australia, 2018.
54. National Health Information and Performance Principal Committee. *The Australian Health Performance Framework*; COAG Health Council: Adelaide, Australia, 2017.
55. Australian Institute of Health and Welfare. Australian Health Performance Framework. Available online: https://www.aihw.gov.au/reports-data/australias-health-performance (accessed on 5 November 2021).
56. Australian Institute of Health and Welfare. *Chronic Conditions and Disability 2015*; Cat. No. CDK 8; AIHW: Canberra, Australia, 2018.
57. Australian Institute of Health and Welfare. *Disability and Its Relationship to Health Conditions and other Factors*; AIHW Cat. No. DIS 37; AIHW: Canberra, Australia, 2004.
58. Australian Institute of Health and Welfare. *Australia's Welfare 2005*; AIHW: Canberra, Australia, 2005.

59. Fortune, N.; Badland, H.; Stancliffe, R.J.; Emerson, E.; Llewellyn, G. *Disability and Wellbeing Monitoring Framework: Baseline Indicator Data for Australians Aged 18–64 Years*; Centre of Research Excellence in Disability and Health: Melbourne, Australia, 2021; (Forthcoming).
60. Fortune, N.; Badland, H.; Clifton, S.; Emerson, E.; Rachele, J.; Stancliffe, R.J.; Zhou, Q.; Llewellyn, G. The Disability and Wellbeing Monitoring Framework: Data, data gaps, and policy implications. *Aust. N. Z. J. Public Health* **2020**, *44*, 227–232. [CrossRef]
61. Canaway, R.; Boyle, D.I.; Manski-Nankervis, J.A.E.; Bell, J.; Hocking, J.S.; Clarke, K.; Clark, M.; Gunn, J.M.; Emery, J.D. Gathering data for decisions: Best practice use of primary care electronic records for research. *Med. J. Aust.* **2019**, *210*, S12–S16. [CrossRef]
62. Bailie, R.; Bailie, J.; Chakraborty, A.; Swift, K. Consistency of denominator data in electronic health records in Australian primary healthcare services: Enhancing data quality. *Aust. J. Prim. Health* **2015**, *21*, 450–459. [CrossRef] [PubMed]
63. Foley, K.-R.; Pollack, A.J.; Britt, H.C.; Lennox, N.G.; Trollor, J.N. General practice encounters for young patients with autism spectrum disorder in Australia. *Autism* **2018**, *22*, 784–793. [CrossRef] [PubMed]
64. Weise, J.; Pollack, A.; Britt, H.; Trollor, J. Primary health care for people with an intellectual disability: An exploration of consultations, problems identified, and their management in Australia. *J. Intellect. Disabil. Res.* **2017**, *61*, 399–410. [CrossRef] [PubMed]
65. Weise, J.; Pollack, A.; Britt, H.; Trollor, J.N. Primary health care for people with an intellectual disability: An exploration of demographic characteristics and reasons for encounters from the BEACH programme. *J. Intellect. Disabil. Res.* **2016**, *60*, 1119–1127. [CrossRef]
66. Reppermund, S.; Heintze, T.; Srasuebkul, P.; Reeve, R.; Dean, K.; Smith, M.; Emerson, E.; Snoyman, P.; Baldry, E.; Dowse, L. Health and wellbeing of people with intellectual disability in New South Wales, Australia: A data linkage cohort. *BMJ Open* **2019**, *9*, e031624. [CrossRef]
67. Reppermund, S.; Srasuebkul, P.; Dean, K.; Trollor, J.N. Factors associated with death in people with intellectual disability. *J. Appl. Res. Intellect. Disabil.* **2020**, *33*, 420–429. [CrossRef]
68. Reppermund, S.; Srasuebkul, P.; Heintze, T.; Reeve, R.; Dean, K.; Emerson, E.; Coyne, D.; Snoyman, P.; Baldry, E.; Dowse, L. Cohort profile: A data linkage cohort to examine health service profiles of people with intellectual disability in New South Wales, Australia. *BMJ Open* **2017**, *7*, e015627. [CrossRef]
69. Florio, T.; Trollor, J. Mortality among a cohort of persons with an intellectual disability in New South Wales, Australia. *J. Appl. Res. Intellect. Disabil.* **2015**, *28*, 383–393. [CrossRef]
70. Balogh, R.; Leonard, H.; Bourke, J.; Brameld, K.; Downs, J.; Hansen, M.; Glasson, E.; Lin, E.; Lloyd, M.; Lunsky, Y. Data linkage: Canadian and Australian perspectives on a valuable methodology for intellectual and developmental disability research. *IDD* **2019**, *57*, 439–462. [CrossRef]
71. Hwang, Y.I.; Srasuebkul, P.; Foley, K.R.; Arnold, S.; Trollor, J.N. Mortality and cause of death of Australians on the autism spectrum. *Autism Res.* **2019**, *12*, 806–815. [CrossRef]
72. Brameld, K.; Spilsbury, K.; Rosenwax, L.; Leonard, H.; Semmens, J. Use of health services in the last year of life and cause of death in people with intellectual disability: A retrospective matched cohort study. *BMJ Open* **2018**, *8*, e020268. [CrossRef]
73. Linton, S. Disability Studies/Not Disability Studies. *Disabil. Soc.* **1998**, *13*, 525–539. [CrossRef]
74. Bruce, C. Unsettling ableism in research traditions: Toward establishing blind methodologies. In *Social Research and Disability*; Routledge: Oxfordshire, UK, 2020; pp. 127–140.
75. Clifton, S.; Fortune, N.; Llewellyn, G.; Stancliffe, R.J.; Williamson, P. Lived expertise and the development of a framework for tracking the social determinants, health, and wellbeing of Australians with disability. *Scand. J. Disabil. Res.* **2020**, *22*, 137–146. [CrossRef]
76. Judith, W.; Gillian, K.; Neil, D.; Katie, W. Indigenous data sovereignty in higher education: Towards a decolonised data quality framework. *Aust. Univ. Rev.* **2018**, *60*, 4–14. [CrossRef]
77. Nind, M. *What Is Inclusive Research?* 1st ed.; What is? Research Methods Series; Bloomsbury Publishing Plc: London, UK, 2014.
78. Bigby, C.; Frawley, P.; Ramcharan, P. Conceptualizing Inclusive Research with People with Intellectual Disability. *J. Appl. Res. Intellect. Disabil.* **2014**, *27*, 3–12. [CrossRef]
79. Roennfeldt, H.; Byrne, L. Lived experience researchers: Opportunities and challenges in mental health. In *Social Research and Disability*; Routledge: Oxfordshire, UK, 2020; pp. 108–123.
80. Dalton, A.J.; McVilly, K.R. Ethics Guidelines for International, Multicenter Research Involving People with Intellectual Disabilities1,2,3,4. *J. Policy Pract. Intellect. Disabil.* **2004**, *1*, 57–70. [CrossRef]
81. McDonald, K.E.; Kidney, C.A. What is right? *Ethics in intellectual disabilities research*. *J. Policy Pract. Intellect. Disabil.* **2012**, *9*, 27–39. [CrossRef]
82. Taua, C.; Neville, C.; Hepworth, J. Research participation by people with intellectual disability and mental health issues: An examination of the processes of consent. *Int. J. Ment. Health Nurs.* **2014**, *23*, 513–524. [CrossRef]
83. McDonald, K.E.; Keys, C.B.; Henry, D.B. Gatekeepers of science: Attitudes toward the research participation of adults with intellectual disability. *Am. J. Ment. Retard.* **2008**, *113*, 466–478. [CrossRef]
84. Mello, A.G.D. Deficiência, incapacidade e vulnerabilidade: Do capacitismo ou a preeminência capacitista e biomédica do Comitê de Ética em Pesquisa da UFSC. *Ciência Saúde Coletiva* **2016**, *21*, 3265–3276. [CrossRef]
85. Sutherland, R.J.; Isherwood, T. The Evidence for easy-read for people with intellectual disabilities: A Systematic Literature Review. *J. Policy Pract. Intellect. Disabil.* **2016**, *13*, 297–310. [CrossRef]

86. McDonald, K.E.; Conroy, N.E.; Olick, R.S.; Panel, T.P.E.E. What's the harm? *Harms in research with adults with intellectual disability. Am. J. Intellect. Dev. Disabil.* **2017**, *122*, 78–92. [CrossRef] [PubMed]
87. Williams, P. 'It all sounds very interesting, but we're just too busy!': Exploring why 'gatekeepers' decline access to potential research participants with learning disabilities. *Eur. J. Spec. Needs Educ.* **2020**, *35*, 1–14. [CrossRef]
88. Baldry, E.; Briggs, D.B.; Goldson, B.; Russell, S. 'Cruel and unusual punishment': An inter-jurisdictional study of the criminalisation of young people with complex support needs. *J. Youth Stud.* **2018**, *21*, 636–652. [CrossRef]
89. Ellem, K.; Wilson, J.; Chui, W.H.; Knox, M. Ethical challenges of life story research with ex-prisoners with intellectual disability. *Disabil. Soc.* **2008**, *23*, 497–509. [CrossRef]
90. Vanny, K.; Levy, M.; Hayes, S. People with an intellectual disability in the Australian criminal justice system. *Psychiatry Psychol. Law* **2008**, *15*, 261–271. [CrossRef]
91. McCausland, R.; Baldry, E. 'I feel like I failed him by ringing the police': Criminalising disability in Australia. *Punishm. Soc.* **2017**, *19*, 290–309. [CrossRef]
92. Temple, J.B.; Wong, H.; Ferdinand, A.; Avery, S.; Paradies, Y.; Kelaher, M. Exposure to interpersonal racism and avoidance behaviours reported by Aboriginal and Torres Strait Islander people with a disability. *Aust. J. Soc. Issues* **2020**, *55*, 376–395. [CrossRef]
93. Avery, S. *Culture is Inclusion: A narrative of Aboriginal and Torres Strait Islander People with Disability*; First Peoples Disability Network: Sydney, Australia, 2018.
94. Walsh, C.; Puszka, S. *Aboriginal and Torres Strait Islander Voices in Disability Support Services: A Collation of Systematic Reviews*; Commissioned Report; Centre for Aboriginal Economic Policy Research, Australian National University: Canberra, Australia, 2021.
95. Australian Institute of Health and Welfare. *A Guide to Data Development*; AIHW Cat. No. HWI 94; AIHW: Canberra, Australia, 2007.
96. World Health Organization; United Nations ESCAP. *Training Manual on Disability Statistics*; United Nations: Bangkok, Thailand, 2008.

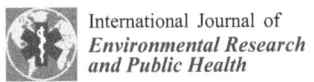

Commentary

General Practice Statistics in Australia: Pushing a Round Peg into a Square Hole

Julie Gordon [1,*], Helena Britt [2], Graeme C. Miller [2], Joan Henderson [2], Anthony Scott [3] and Christopher Harrison [4]

[1] WHO Collaborating Centre for Strengthening Rehabilitation Capacity in Health Systems, University of Sydney, Sydney, NSW 2006, Australia

[2] Sydney School of Public Health, University of Sydney, Sydney, NSW 2006, Australia; helena.britt@sydney.edu.au (H.B.); graeme.miller@sydney.edu.au (G.C.M.); joan.henderson@sydney.edu.au (J.H.)

[3] Melbourne Institute of Applied Economic and Social Research, University of Melbourne, Melbourne, VIC 3053, Australia; a.scott@unimelb.edu.au

[4] Menzies Centre for Health Policy and Economics, Sydney School of Public Health, University of Sydney, Sydney, NSW 2006, Australia; christopher.harrison@sydney.edu.au

* Correspondence: julie.gordon@sydney.edu.au

Abstract: In Australia, general practice forms a core part of the health system, with general practitioners (GPs) having a gatekeeper role for patients to receive care from other health services. GPs manage the care of patients across their lifespan and have roles in preventive health care, chronic condition management, multimorbidity and population health. Most people in Australia see a GP once in any given year. Draft reforms have been released by the Australian Government that may change the model of general practice currently implemented in Australia. In order to quantify the impact and effectiveness of any implemented reforms in the future, reliable and valid data about general practice clinical activity over time, will be needed. In this context, this commentary outlines the historical and current approaches used to obtain general practice statistics in Australia and highlights the benefits and limitations of these approaches. The role of data generated from GP electronic health record extractions is discussed. A methodology to generate high quality statistics from Australian general practice in the future is presented.

Keywords: general practice; health services research; primary health care

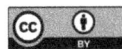

1. Introduction

General practice is the foundation of the Australian healthcare system, as general practitioners (GPs) are the gatekeepers for patient access to many other health services. Reliable data about GP clinical activity is needed for statistical analysis by primary care and public health researchers, those involved with health policy, health services planning and costing, GP educators, health consumers, and those involved in the development and production of health treatments and interventions. In this commentary article we will discuss the historical and current approaches used to obtain statistics in Australian general practice, highlight benefits and limitations in these approaches, and outline a proposed methodology to generate high quality statistics from general practice in the future.

2. Background

General practice forms a core part of the Australian healthcare system, often representing a patient's initial contact with the system. GPs in Australia manage patients across their lifespan, manage chronic health conditions and multimorbidity, and provide preventive healthcare. They also have a 'gatekeeper' role, providing referrals for patients to access other services including care from non-GP specialists, and subsidized care from allied health professionals for patients with chronic conditions. Currently, patients are free to attend one or more GPs of their choice, and are not assigned to a particular GP or practice. While patients have this freedom, most attend the same practice for continuity of care ([1], Chapter 15). In Australia, general practices are usually private medical practices providing "comprehensive, coordinated and continuing medical care drawing on biomedical, psychological, social and environmental understandings of health" [2].

In 2019, there were over 37,000 GPs in Australia, working across 8147 general practices [3].

According to data from the World Bank, 86% of the Australian population lived in urban areas in 2020 [4], primarily along the East Coast. Accordingly, in 2019, approximately three-quarters (74.5%) of full-time equivalent GPs reported working in major cities [3]. In any one year, approximately 87% of the population see a GP, and on average, there were six GP visits per head of population in Australia in 2015–2016 [1].

In March 2021, Australia had a population of 25.7 million people [5]. Funding of health services in Australia is the responsibility of the federal (national) and state/territory (regional) governments. Spending on health totaled $197.7 billion (Australian) dollars in 2018–2019, equating to $7772 per head of population [6]. Health spending represented 10% of gross domestic product.

In 2018–2019 $65.5 billion was spent on primary health care [6], which incorporated general practice, allied and community health, and pharmacy (excluding Indigenous health care). General practice is primarily funded by the federal government on a 'fee for service' model, where GPs can charge any fee they wish, and patients receive a fixed subsidy according to the Medicare Benefits Schedule (MBS), a catalogue of medical services for which a rebate can be claimed from the government [7]. If the fee for a consultation or service provided is equal to the Medicare subsidy, then the consultation is 'bulk billed'. Around 87% of GP services are bulk-billed [3]. If not, then the patient pays an out-of-pocket cost decided by the GP. For patients with very high out-of-pocket costs for GP and non-GP specialist consultations, additional subsidies are provided through the Medicare Safety Net [8]. Medicare items for GP consultations are based on broad estimates of consultation length and complexity. Limited items are related to specific diseases or for specific population groups (e.g., annual health assessments for patients aged 75+ years, or chronic disease management plans for patients with diabetes). Other Medicare-rebatable services include pathology tests, imaging tests and procedures undertaken. A separate Pharmaceutical Benefits Scheme (PBS) provides public subsidies for most prescribed medications dispensed by pharmacists [9].

The important role of general practice within the wider healthcare system has been recognized for some time. White et al. introduced a framework in Britain in 1961 to depict the organization of health care, demonstrating that within a population of 1000 adults, 250 (or 25%) will consult a physician (i.e., a primary care doctor or GP) in any one month. Nine of these 250 patients seeking care will be hospitalized, and five referred to another physician for care [10]. The overall stability of this framework has been established over time [11,12]. The aim of generating statistics from general practice is therefore not only to understand clinical activity undertaken in this setting, but to understand the health of the population overall.

In August 2019, the Australian Government released 'Australia's long-term national health plan'. The plan contained four 'pillars' (focus areas), the first of which was to strengthen the role of primary health care in the Australian healthcare system [13]. Later that year, a Primary Healh Reform Steering Group was established, focusing on the development of a ten-year plan for primary health care [14]. The draft report for the 'Primary Health Care 10 Year Plan' was released in October 2021 for consultation. The draft reforms are wide-ranging, containing changes to the funding models used in general practice, methods of general practice care delivery, and the introduction of patient registration at a single GP practice. The need for data to guide policy and quality improvement is reinforced in the plan [15].

If the draft reforms are implemented, there will likely be a multitude of changes to the current model of general practice in Australia. The proposed introduction of patient registration at a GP practice might further the role of the GP as central to population health. High-quality evidence-based statistics are required, to establish a baseline dataset for current general practice care delivery, and to assess the impact and effectiveness of any implemented reforms. This presents a timely opportunity to review the current state of general practice statistics in Australia.

3. History of General Practice Statistics in Australia

A detailed history of general practice data collection and analysis in Australia has been described elsewhere [16]. The first general practice survey was conducted by Dr Clifford Jungfer (GP) and Dr John Last (epidemiologist) in 1959–1960, with support from the (then) Australian College of General Practitioners [17]. This was followed by a National Morbidity Survey in 1962 [18]. Meanwhile, Dr Kevin Cullen, a GP in the town of Busselton, Western Australia, began the Busselton Health Study, a longitudinal study of population groups within Busselton conducted between 1966 and 1981. The Busselton Health Study was based on repeated cross-sectional surveys comprising questionnaires and blood tests to investigate the health of the study population, and identify health indicators that predicted future disease [19].

The Australian General Practice Morbidity and Prescribing Survey was conducted from 1969 to 1974, started by the Royal Australian College of General Practitioners' research committee, and led by Dr Charles Bridges-Webb [20]. The methods used in this study became the foundation for subsequent surveys of general practice clinical activity, including the Australian Morbidity and Treatment Survey (1990–1991) [21] and the Bettering the Evaluation and Care of Health (BEACH) study (1998–2016) [1].

For 18 years, the BEACH study described the clinical activity undertaken by GPs in Australia [1]. In BEACH, 1000 randomly selected GPs were sampled in each year of the study. Each GP participant recorded de-identified data for about 100 consecutive patient encounters on structured paper forms. Data collected included some patient demographics (e.g., date of birth, patient sex, postcode, Indigeneity), the patients' reasons for encounter (up to three), problems managed at the encounter (up to 4), medications prescribed/supplied/advised for purchase, for each problem, other treatments provided for each problem (including procedures and clinical treatments, such as advice and counselling), and pathology and imaging requests for each problem. Importantly, each management action was explicitly linked to the problem for which that action was taken. More detailed methods for the BEACH study can be found elsewhere [1]. BEACH closed in 2016 due to the withdrawal of support from the federal government (both funding and loss of the random samples of GPs provided) and wider losses of research support from industry partners [16]. With a final database spanning 18 years and approximately 1.8 million GP–patient encounter records, BEACH data were used to investigate the problems managed by GPs, how GPs managed these problems during consultations, and how the quality of care provided by GPs compared to evidence-based guidelines. BEACH data also identified changes in general practice clinical activity over time [22] and provided evidence about numerous policy areas, including time spent on patient care not able to be claimed through the MBS [23], the potential cost of freezing MBS item rebates [24] and (using length of consultation data) disproved statements that GPs were providing so-called 'six minute medicine' [25]. It was widely recognized that the closure of BEACH created a gap in data available about general practice [26]. Irving et al., in their investigation of primary care physician consultation time, presented a rather thorough international comparison of general practice data collection methods through their systematic review of 67 countries, and concluded that the Australian BEACH study "represents the gold standard for consistent reporting" [27].

The end of BEACH coincided with the closure of a number of other sources of data about general practice in Australia. Government funding was withdrawn from the Australian Primary Health Care Research Institute in 2015 [28]. The Medicine in Australia: Balancing Employment and Life (MABEL) study, a longitudinal study about the medical workforce, ended in 2019, after 11 waves of data collection. This study provided numerous insights on access to medical care from between 3000 and 4000 GPs, followed up each year, including the drivers of hours worked, job satisfaction, and factors influencing recruitment and retention in rural areas [29]. The Australian Government's Medical Research Future Fund, established to provide grants for health and medical research, is reported to allocate less than 1% of total funding to primary care research [30]. Currently, many gaps exist in the statistics available from general practice, both in terms of the data collected and the research conducted [31].

4. Current Status of General Practice Clinical Activity Data

Limited administrative data are available about general practice from the MBS and the PBS. The MBS has records of the consultation items claimed by GPs from Government, but these provide very limited understanding of the clinical content of the consultation or the characteristics of the GPs. Similarly, the PBS contains data about subsidized medications dispensed by pharmacies, but does not include data about the clinical indication (i.e., symptom or diagnosis) for which the medication was prescribed. To obtain data about the clinical content of GP consultations, we need to look elsewhere.

General practice was one of the early adopters of computerized clinical records, with government incentives to use computers available as early as 1998 [32]. Computerization began in the early 1990s, and some of the early systems developed (e.g., Medical Director) are still commonly used today [33]. There are now at least eight brands of electronic health records (EHRs) currently used in Australian general practice [33]. According to BEACH data, in 2014–2015, 97.5 % of Australian GPs reported that they used a computer for one or more purposes. However, only 70.7% used paperless medical records while 25.5% used hybrid (paper and electronic) records [22]. The MABEL survey in 2018 also asked about GPs' use of digital technology for a range of tasks, and found (for example) almost 90% of GPs using digital technology to view imaging pathology and results [34]. These data demonstrate that while GPs have a high uptake of computerized medical records and digital technologies, some still rely on paper for some activities.

While the BEACH study was conducted on paper, some GPs said they would have preferred to be able to download data from their practice electronic health records (EHRs) to be used in the study. There were two primary reasons that structured paper forms were used in BEACH. First, to facilitate the linkages between the problems managed and all management actions provided for each problem. The problem–management linkage in BEACH ensured the GP specifically linked the prescription of a medication to the problem for which it was prescribed. It remains extremely difficult, if not impossible, to obtain these linkages from EHR data. This has led some researchers, using GP EHR data, to secondarily link each medication to a problem in the record on the basis of 'probability'. However, medications will often have multiple possible indications, let alone other off-label uses, making it difficult to know what health problem it is treating, and making matching by assumption highly unreliable. Second, BEACH was a study of GP clinical activity. The structured paper forms were inherently transportable, so that GPs who worked in multiple practices could take the forms between practices, or to home visits or nursing home visits. Secondary data entry by trained clinical coders, while time consuming and costly, facilitated consistent coding of the data to improve data quality.

In the absence of BEACH data since 2016, statistics from general practice have become focused on data extracted from EHRs. There are numerous research programs in Australia that rely on de-identified data extracted from GP EHRs, including:

(1) MedicineInsight (NPS MedicineWise);
(2) Data for Decisions (University of Melbourne);
(3) Primary Health Insights (led by WA Primary Health Alliance).

Data extraction from EHRs may be as basic as a simple export tool. More complex extraction tools have been developed specifically for this purpose [35], for example GRHANITE (University of Melbourne) [36], the CAT4 tool (Pen Computing) [37] and

POLAR GP [38]. These tools can be used at multiple levels—for clinical audit or quality improvement activities at the practice, or by the local health region (called Primary Health Networks or PHNs in Australia), or to provide data to research programs at a wider level.

5. The Use of EHR Data for Research and Statistics

The automated extraction of data already collected during the clinical patient encounter creates a database of 'passive' data that can be used for statistics and research. While the primary purpose of data collection in an EHR is for patient care, making these data available for research and statistics minimizes the effort for individual GPs (who are often poor in time [39,40]) to participate in studies for multiple research groups. However, organizing and performing data extraction does involve time and effort for the practice. GPs report that it is often practice staff who undertake these activities [40], so the process is not entirely automated and does have a cost, although this is not always perceived as a barrier [41].

Passively collected data creates large volumes of data that can be interrogated in many ways. This provides greater scope to examine the management of rare phenomena. Theoretically, for patients who regularly attend the same practice, EHR data extraction allows for the longitudinal analysis of a patient's journey over time, providing the potential to assess medical interventions and long-term health outcomes. This is limited though, if patients attend multiple practices (e.g., while travelling or for convenience) or change practices for any reason, resulting in incomplete data.

5.1. Variability in EHR Design

Interoperability of data requires standard approaches to data design structures, data field names and their associated definitions, and the coding and classification of relevant data fields. Standardization is required to enable data to be combined from different EHRs for clinical audits and research, and to facilitate the transfer of patient care between different healthcare providers (e.g., referrals). All of the GP EHRs used in Australia have been developed independently, which limits such interoperability and the ability to generate meaningful data from general practice EHRs, both for clinical and statistical purposes [33,35].

There are differences in the underlying designs of the EHR database structures, including the data field names, their definitions, and how data fields are or are not linked. There are also vast inconsistencies in the use of clinical classifications and terminologies, including the type of clinical terminology used (e.g., termsets developed by individual EHR developers, ICPC-2 PLUS [42] or SNOMED CT-AU [43]). In most EHRs, clinicians can choose whether to enter a term from one of these termsets or to enter free text [33]. As a result, most EHR research databases extract data from only some of the available EHRs, limiting the representativeness of the data. For example, MedicineInsight extracts data from the two most commonly used EHRs [44], each of which uses a different coding system.

5.2. Data Completeness

The quality of research and statistics is only ever as good as the quality of the data contained in the record from which the data are extracted. Data accuracy in EHRs has been found to be variable [35,41], which is likely to impact on research quality. In one recent Australian study, approximately 13% of probable cases did not have a coded diagnosis, and were identified through the presence of one or more other diabetes management indicators [45].

Bailie et al. (2015) identified difficulties in calculating denominators in patient data extracted from EHRs. Numerous reasons were given, including incomplete data entry, differing requirements and compatibility between EHRs and data extraction tools, and differences in the definition used for active or regular patients. The authors concluded that the inconsistencies identified limited the usefulness and reliability of the EHR data [46].

5.3. The Medical Record as an 'Aide Memoir'

The primary purpose of the EHR is to capture data that relates to the clinical care of the patient, not to obtain data for research purposes [47]. Henderson et al. (2019) suggest that time-poor GPs may only enter the data they regard as important for patient care, which may not always reflect the data that are important for research. This limits the capability of using EHR data for research purposes [45].

The medical record has long been regarded as an 'aide memoir', or memory aid, rather than as a complete record of the patient's care. Even with the advent of EHRs, this association has continued. In a benchmarking study that examined the prevalence of diabetes using BEACH data and extracted data from one Australian EHR, the prevalence of diabetes was lower when using the extracted EHR data from the 'diagnosis' data element. However, the authors found that they could obtain a comparable prevalence estimate by identifying proxies that indicate the presence of diabetes (e.g., free text searches for diabetes in other parts of the record, medications used to treat diabetes, use of MBS item numbers only used in relation to diabetes). Importantly, the authors noted that this approach would be less reliable for other clinical conditions where proxy measures may not work [45]. Interestingly, MedicineInsight does not extract free text data, as it may contain identifiable information that could compromise privacy [44].

5.4. Privacy and Information Protection

The extraction of data from EHRs for statistical and research purposes usually involves the transfer of the exported patient data to a third party (e.g., government department or University researcher). Concerns have arisen in Australia about patient privacy and information protection [35,40,41]. The removal of information from extracted data that would identify a patient has been highlighted as being of primary importance to researchers [35,41,48], GPs [40,41] and other practice staff [41]. The need for independent governance oversight of programs that involve extracted EHR data has also been emphasized [35,48].

At present, most data extraction from general practice EHRs involves the whole of practice data, where data are extracted about all patient encounters [44]. Concerns may arise if individual GPs within a practice are not willing to have data about their clinical activity included in a download, or when patients do not give permission for their data to be downloaded.

6. A Fresh Approach

We propose a new approach to improve the production of high-quality data about general practice clinical activity. This proposal is based on the following principles:

(1) Data from general practice can provide an excellent overview of the health of the population overall;
(2) Using the GP as an 'expert interviewer' to curate data can facilitate data with higher levels of accuracy than patient self-report;
(3) It is not necessary to collect data about all the patients, all the time. The BEACH study demonstrated that the production of structured data, about a sample of patients, can generate high-quality statistics from general practice for use in policy planning, education, and research;
(4) The sample of patients must be representative of the patient population to ensure validity and reliability;
(5) Data need to be longitudinal for the investigation of outcomes of care, including care provided by other health services (e.g., specialists, hospitals);
(6) The capacity to review the patient's experience with the health system overall, through linking general practice data to that from other health agencies, is encouraged.

Building on the structure of the BEACH interface for active data collection, we propose developing a hybrid active + passive data collection based on data extraction from EHRs with subsequent data curation from GPs to review the quality of extracted data and complete gaps in the dataset. A specialized data extraction tool would be required to extract relevant data from the GP EHR. To circumvent problems experienced with current EHR data extractions, the GP would curate the data for completeness and validity.

We propose that two data templates are required:

(1) A health summary template where the GP extracts a health summary from the EHR (similar to the patient summary currently contained in the EHR), followed by a 'check and curate' process, in which the GP reviews the accuracy and completeness of the data extracted. For example, is the patient's problem list accurate? Are medications listed that the patient no longer takes, or are there over-the-counter medications taken regularly that should be added? There are also additional data elements not currently included in GP EHRs that could be captured in this process. For example, capture of data about social determinants of health (e.g., education level, household income) would contribute to a greater understanding of a patient's health and related health outcomes;

(2) An encounter summary template where the GP extracts and curates data about an individual GP–patient encounter. This data extraction would be based on data elements that were collected in BEACH using a problem-oriented structure. The GP would curate the data by completing areas within the template that are missing and add linkages between problems managed and their treatments.

For each of these, minimum datasets based on a problem-oriented record structure with in-built coding and classification systems would be required for the purposes of data extraction, encryption and transfer to researchers, and subsequent data analysis.

Initially, these could be used to provide cross-sectional data from a representative sample of patients who attend general practice. A second stage of research would involve use of the tool as the basis for longitudinal data collection, whereby a sample of patients are recruited to the study and their data are extracted and curated at every visit. The addition of data about other health services received between GP visits (e.g., specialist, hospital or allied health visits), added and curated by the GP, would enhance knowledge about patients' broader experiences with the health system.

The strength of this approach is the focus placed on the importance of record structures, data linkages, coding and classification systems, and in the general application of standards required for the success of the model.

This approach will improve the understanding of morbidity and management within the general practice population and provide baseline data for further research and evaluation examining interventions to improve quality of care for general practice patients. It has some utility for use in GP clinical audits and quality assurance.

7. Conclusions

The Primary Health Care Reforms currently under consideration reference the 'quadruple aim' of health care, improving: (1) people's experiences with health care; (2) population health; (3) cost-efficiency of the health system; and (4) work life for healthcare workers [49]. The first three of these are quantifiable measures that rely on the availability of relevant data, and statistical analysis of these data, to assess the effectiveness of any reforms implemented to achieve these aims.

There is a reliance on data currently contained in GP EHRs to answer these questions, as shown in the reform policy and in initiatives such as the Australian Institute of Health and Welfare's Primary Health Care Data Asset. Current forms of data extraction from EHRs might be economically preferable and can answer some questions, but they cannot answer all of them. The temptation to use these datasets may equate to 'trying to fit a square peg into a round hole', an idiom that implies a solution that is unfit for purpose. Rather than accepting or ignoring the limitations of EHR data that currently exist, why not be aspirational? How can we achieve better statistics from general practice that are able to inform both the patient and provider experience, and can be used for system planning?

COVID-19 has changed the way general practice services are conducted in Australia. The availability [50] and use [51] of telehealth services represents a dramatic shift in the way general practice services are provided to the public. However, there are little data available about how COVID-19 has changed the clinical activity undertaken by GPs and the quality of care provided through telehealth. Changes to the GP workforce resulting from COVID-19, and the future intentions of the GP workforce may have also been impacted by the pandemic, but with little data available it is impossible to quantify these. The approach presented in this paper for improving clinical activity data should be complemented by reinvestment in longitudinal data about the GP workforce, lost by the cessation of the MABEL study.

The approach to general practice data outlined in this paper may not answer every question that could be asked about general practice, but it would go a long way in overcoming the current deficiencies, and would produce national, valid, reliable statistics from Australian general practice.

Author Contributions: Conceptualization, J.G., H.B., G.C.M., J.H. and C.H.; investigation, J.G., H.B., G.C.M., J.H., A.S. and C.H.; writing—original draft, J.G., H.B. and G.C.M.; writing—review and editing, J.G., H.B., G.C.M., J.H., A.S. and C.H. All authors have read and agreed to the published version of the manuscript.

Funding: This research received no external funding.

Institutional Review Board Statement: Not applicable.

Informed Consent Statement: Not applicable.

Data Availability Statement: Not applicable.

Conflicts of Interest: The authors declare no conflict of interest.

References

1. Britt, H.; Miller, G.C.; Henderson, J.; Bayram, C.; Harrison, C.; Valenti, L.; Pan, Y.; Charles, J.; Pollack, A.J.; Wong, C. *General Practice Activity in Australia 2015–16*; Sydney University Press: Sydney, Australia, 2016.
2. Royal Australian College of General Practitioners. General Practice Training Terms and Definitions. Available online: https://www.racgp.org.au/education/gps/supervisors-and-examiners/supervising-medical-students/definitions (accessed on 18 January 2022).
3. Australian Government Productivity Commission. Report on Government Services 2021: 10 Primary and Community Health. Available online: https://www.pc.gov.au/research/ongoing/report-on-government-services/2021/health/primary-and-community-health (accessed on 10 November 2021).
4. The World Bank. Urban Population (% of Total Population)-Australia. Available online: https://data.worldbank.org/indicator/SP.URB.TOTL.IN.ZS?locations=AU (accessed on 10 November 2021).
5. Australian Bureau of Statistics. National, State and Territory Population. Available online: https://www.abs.gov.au/statistics/people/population/national-state-and-territory-population/mar-2021 (accessed on 9 November 2021).
6. Australian Institute of Health and Welfare. *Health Expenditure Australia 2018–19. Health and Welfare Expenditure Series*; No.66. Cat. No. HWE 80; AIHW: Canberra, Australia, 2020.
7. Australian Government Department of Health. MBS Online 04/21. Available online: http://www.mbsonline.gov.au/internet/mbsonline/publishing.nsf/Content/Home (accessed on 20 September 2020).
8. Australian Government-Services Australia. Medicare Safety Nets. Available online: https://www.servicesaustralia.gov.au/medicare-safety-nets (accessed on 13 December 2021).
9. Pearson, S.-A.; Pratt, N.; de Oliveira Costa, J.; Zoega, H.; Laba, T.-L.; Etherton-Beer, C.; Sanfilippo, F.M.; Morgan, A.; Kalisch Ellett, L.; Bruno, C. Generating Real-World Evidence on the Quality Use, Benefits and Safety of Medicines in Australia: History, Challenges and a Roadmap for the Future. *Int. J. Environ. Res. Public Health* **2021**, *18*, 13345. [CrossRef] [PubMed]
10. White, K.L.; Williams, T.F.; Greenberg, B.G. The ecology of medical care. 1961. *Bull. N. Y. Acad. Med.* **1996**, *73*, 187. [PubMed]
11. Green, L.A.; Fryer, G.E., Jr.; Yawn, B.P.; Lanier, D.; Dovey, S.M. The Ecology of Medical Care Revisited. *N. Engl. J. Med.* **2001**, *344*, 2021–2025. Available online: https://10.1056/NEJM200106283442611 (accessed on 15 November 2021). [CrossRef] [PubMed]
12. Johansen, M.E.; Kircher, S.M.; Huerta, T.R. Reexamining the ecology of medical care. *N. Engl. J. Med.* **2016**, *374*, 495–496. [CrossRef]
13. Australian Government Department of Health. *Australia's Long Term National Health Plan to Build the World's Best Health System*; Department of Health: Canberra, Australia, 2019.

14. Australian Government Department of Health. Primary Health Care Reform. Available online: https://www1.health.gov.au/internet/main/publishing.nsf/Content/primary-health-care-reform (accessed on 14 November 2021).
15. Australian Government Department of Health. *Consultation Draft-Future Focused Primary Health Care: Australia's Primary Health Care 10 Year Plan 2022–2032*; Department of Health: Canberra, Australia, 2021.
16. Britt, H.; Miller, G.C. Measuring general practice activity in Australia: A brief history. *Aust. Fam. Physician* **2017**, *46*, 343–345.
17. Jungfer, C.; Last, J. Clinical performance in Australian general practice. *Med. Care* **1964**, *2*, 71–83. [CrossRef]
18. National Health and Medical Research Council. *Report on a National Morbidity Survey Part 1*; NHMRC: Canberra, Australia, 1966.
19. Busselton Population Medical Research Institute. Busselton Health Study-History. Available online: http://bpmri.org.au/about-us/history/busselton-health-study-history.html (accessed on 15 November 2021).
20. Bridges-Webb, C. The Australian general practice morbidity and prescribing survey, 1969 to 1974. *Med. J. Aust.* **1976**, *2*, 1–28.
21. Bridges-Webb, C.; Britt, H.; Miles, D.; Neary, S.; Charles, J. Morbidity and treatment in general practice in Australia 1990–1991. *Med. J. Aust.* **1992**, *157*, S1–S56. [CrossRef]
22. Britt, H.; Miller, G.C.; Bayram, C.; Henderson, J.; Valenti, L.; Harrison, C.; Pan, Y.; Charles, J.; Pollack, A.J.; Chambers, T. *A Decade of Australian General Practice Activity 2006–07 to 2015–16*; Sydney University Press: Sydney, Australia, 2016.
23. Henderson, J.; Valenti, L.A.; Britt, H.C.; Bayram, C.; Wong, C.; Harrison, C.; Pollack, A.J.; Gordon, J.; Miller, G.C. Estimating non-billable time in Australian general practice. *Med. J. Aust.* **2016**, *205*, 79–83. [CrossRef]
24. Harrison, C.; Bayram, C.; Miller, G.C.; Britt, H.C. The cost of freezing general practice. *Med. J. Aust.* **2015**, *202*, 313–316. [CrossRef]
25. Britt, H.; Valenti, L.; Miller, G. Byte from BEACH. No: 2014; 2. Debunking the Myth that General Practice is '6 Minute Medicine'. Available online: https://citeseerx.ist.psu.edu/viewdoc/download?doi=10.1.1.668.7183&rep=rep1&type=pdf (accessed on 15 November 2021).
26. Australian Institute of Health and Welfare. *Developing a National Primary Health Care Data Asset: Consultation Report*; Cat. No. PHC 1; AIHW: Canberra, Australia, 2019.
27. Irving, G.; Neves, A.L.; Dambha-Miller, H.; Oishi, A.; Tagashira, H.; Verho, A.; Holden, J. International variations in primary care physician consultation time: A systematic review of 67 countries. *BMJ Open* **2017**, *7*, e017902. [CrossRef] [PubMed]
28. Winzenberg, T.M.; Gill, G.F. Prioritising general practice research. *Med. J. Aust.* **2016**, *205*, 55–57. [CrossRef] [PubMed]
29. Russell, G.M.; McGrail, M.R.; O'Sullivan, B.; Scott, A. Improving knowledge and data about the medical workforce underpins healthy communities and doctors. *Med. J. Aust.* **2021**, *214*, 252–254.e1. [CrossRef]
30. Hendrie, D. New Wave of GP-Researchers Set to Tackle Vital Questions. Available online: https://www1.racgp.org.au/newsgp/racgp/new-wave-of-gp-researchers-set-to-tackle-vital-que (accessed on 10 December 2021).
31. Tran, B.; Straka, P.; Falster, M.O.; Douglas, K.A.; Britz, T.; Jorm, L.R. Overcoming the data drought: Exploring general practice in Australia by network analysis of big data. *Med. J. Aust.* **2018**, *209*, 68–73. [CrossRef]
32. Commonwealth Department of Health and Aged Care. *General Practice in Australia: 2000*; DHAC: Canberra, Australia, 2000.
33. Gordon, J.; Miller, G.; Britt, H. Reality Check-Reliable National Data from General Practice Electronic Health Records. Available online: https://ahha.asn.au/publication/issue-briefs/deeble-institute-issues-brief-no-18-reality-check-reliable-national-data (accessed on 29 August 2021).
34. Zaresani, A.; Scott, A. Does digital health technology improve physicians' job satisfaction and work–life balance? A cross-sectional national survey and regression analysis using an instrumental variable. *BMJ Open* **2020**, *10*, e041690. [CrossRef] [PubMed]
35. Youens, D.; Moorin, R.; Harrison, A.; Varhol, R.; Robinson, S.; Brooks, C.; Boyd, J. Using general practice clinical information system data for research: The case in Australia. *Int J Popul Data Sci.* **2020**, *5*, 1099. [CrossRef]
36. The University of Melbourne. GRHANITE (TM) Health Informatics Unit. Available online: https://grhanite.unimelb.edu.au/ (accessed on 13 December 2021).
37. PENCS. CAT4. Available online: https://www.pencs.com.au/products/cat4/ (accessed on 13 December 2021).
38. POLAR. POLAR. Cloud-Based Clinical Intelligence. Available online: https://polargp.org.au/ (accessed on 13 December 2021).
39. Brodaty, H.; Gibson, L.H.; Waine, M.L.; Shell, A.M.; Lilian, R.; Pond, C.D. Research in general practice: A survey of incentives and disincentives for research participation. *Ment. Health Fam. Med.* **2013**, *10*, 163. [PubMed]
40. Hodgkins, A.J.; Mullan, J.; Mayne, D.J.; Boyages, C.S.; Bonney, A. Australian general practitioners' attitudes to the extraction of research data from electronic health records. *Aust. J. Gen. Pract.* **2020**, *49*, 145–150. [CrossRef]
41. Monaghan, T.; Manski-Nankervis, J.-A.; Canaway, R. Big data or big risk: General practitioner, practice nurse and practice manager attitudes to providing de-identified patient health data from electronic medical records to researchers. *Aust. J. Prim. Health* **2021**, *26*, 466–471. [CrossRef]
42. The University of Sydney. ICPC-2 PLUS. Available online: https://www.sydney.edu.au/medicine-health/our-research/research-centres/who-collaborating-centre-for-strengthening-rehabilitation-capacity-in-health-systems/classifications-and-terminologies/icpc-2-plus.html (accessed on 13 December 2021).
43. Australian Digital Health Agency. National Clinical Terminology Service. SNOMED CT-AU. Available online: https://www.healthterminologies.gov.au/learn/clinical-terminology/snomed-ct-au/ (accessed on 13 December 2021).
44. Busingye, D.; Gianacas, C.; Pollack, A.; Chidwick, K.; Merrifield, A.; Norman, S.; Mullin, B.; Hayhurst, R.; Blogg, S.; Havard, A. Data Resource Profile: MedicineInsight, an Australian national primary health care database. *Int. J. Epidemiol.* **2019**, *48*, 1741–1741h. [CrossRef]

45. Henderson, J.; Barnett, S.; Ghosh, A.; Pollack, A.J.; Hodgkins, A.; Win, K.T.; Miller, G.C.; Bonney, A. Validation of electronic medical data: Identifying diabetes prevalence in general practice. *Health Inf. Manag. J.* **2019**, *48*, 3–11. [CrossRef] [PubMed]
46. Bailie, R.; Bailie, J.; Chakraborty, A.; Swift, K. Consistency of denominator data in electronic health records in Australian primary healthcare services: Enhancing data quality. *Aust. J. Prim. Health* **2015**, *21*, 450–459. [CrossRef] [PubMed]
47. Barnett, S.; Henderson, J.; Hodgkins, A.; Harrison, C.; Ghosh, A.; Dijkmans-Hadley, B.; Britt, H.; Bonney, A. A valuable approach to the use of electronic medical data in primary care research: Panning for gold. *Health Inf. Manag. J.* **2017**, *46*, 51–57. [CrossRef] [PubMed]
48. Canaway, R.; Boyle, D.I.; Manski-Nankervis, J.A.E.; Bell, J.; Hocking, J.S.; Clarke, K.; Clark, M.; Gunn, J.M.; Emery, J.D. Gathering data for decisions: Best practice use of primary care electronic records for research. *Med. J. Aust.* **2019**, *210*, S12–S16. [CrossRef]
49. Bodenheimer, T.; Sinsky, C. From triple to quadruple aim: Care of the patient requires care of the provider. *Ann. Fam. Med.* **2014**, *12*, 573–576. [CrossRef]
50. Australian Government Department of Health. COVID-19 Temporary MBS Telehealth Services. Section 16 July 2021. Available online: http://www.mbsonline.gov.au/internet/mbsonline/publishing.nsf/Content/Factsheet-TempBB (accessed on 30 September 2021).
51. Scott, A.; Bai, T.; Zhang, Y. Association between telehealth use and general practitioner characteristics during COVID-19: Findings from a nationally representative survey of Australian doctors. *BMJ Open* **2021**, *11*, e046857. [CrossRef]

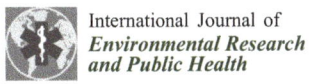

Review

Data Linkage in Australia: The First 50 Years

Merran Smith * and Felicity Flack

Population Health Research Network, University of Western Australia, 35 Stirling Highway, Crawley 6009, Australia; felicity.flack@uwa.edu.au
* Correspondence: merran.smith@uwa.edu.au

Abstract: Population-based data linkage has a long history in Australia from its beginnings in Western Australia in the 1970s to the coordinated national data linkage infrastructure that exists today. This article describes the journey from an idea to a national data linkage network which has impacts on the health and well-being of Australians from preventing developmental anomalies to responding to the COVID-19 pandemic. Many enthusiastic and dedicated people have contributed to Australia's data linkage capability over the last 50 years. They have managed to overcome a number of challenges including gaining stakeholder and community support; navigating complex legal and ethical environments; establishing cross-jurisdictional collaborations, and gaining ongoing financial support. The future is bright for linked data in Australia as the infrastructure built over the last 50 years provides a firm foundation for further expansion and development, ensuring that Australia's linked health and human services data continues to be available to address the evolving challenges of the next half century.

Keywords: data linkage; Australia; cross-jurisdiction

Citation: Smith, M.; Flack, F. Data Linkage in Australia: The First 50 Years. *Int. J. Environ. Res. Public Health* **2021**, *18*, 11339. https://doi.org/10.3390/ijerph182111339

Academic Editor: Richard Madden

Received: 23 September 2021
Accepted: 26 October 2021
Published: 28 October 2021

Publisher's Note: MDPI stays neutral with regard to jurisdictional claims in published maps and institutional affiliations.

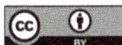

Copyright: © 2021 by the authors. Licensee MDPI, Basel, Switzerland. This article is an open access article distributed under the terms and conditions of the Creative Commons Attribution (CC BY) license (https://creativecommons.org/licenses/by/4.0/).

1. Introduction

Data linkage is a method of bringing together information derived from different sources, but relating to the same individual or event in a single file [1]. It is not a new method; in fact, it predates the introduction of modern computers [1]. For example, in the late 18th century, Edward Jenner conducted what is thought to be the first data linkage, which provided evidence of the efficacy of smallpox vaccination [2].

The term "record linkage" first appeared in the literature in the 20th century in an article by Dr Halbert Dunn, the head of the United States National Office of Vital Statistics, in 1946. In this article, Dunn provides an eloquent description of data linkage and the value of linked data systems.

"Each person in the world creates a Book of Life. This Book starts with birth and ends with death. Its pages are made up of the records of the principal events in life. Record linkage is the name given to the process of assembling the pages of this Book into a volume" [3].

The advent of more advanced mathematical matching techniques and computer technology has enabled the expansion of the use of linked data for population-wide research. It has enabled research across populations and across the life course. Data linkage has become an essential tool in the ongoing understanding and improvement of health and social services worldwide. Linked data is used to:

- Assess outcomes of clinical or therapeutic interventions;
- Assess the safety, quality and costs of health care and other government services;
- Explore the relationships between personal, economic, environmental and lifestyle factors;
- Investigate social and community influences on individual and community health and well-being;
- Assess the effectiveness of preventative programs;

- Obtain valuable follow-up information on participants in research studies and surveys [4].

Whilst the benefits of data linkage can be clearly demonstrated, there are also risks. Linking data and the analysis of linked data requires the use of person-level data often without informed consent. This means that data linkage operates within complex legal and ethical frameworks designed to protect and balance the multiple interests at play. The history of data linkage is infused with the challenges associated with balancing the benefits against the risks to individuals and groups.

Australia has been at the forefront of the uses of linked data and development of linkage systems for more than fifty years. It is timely to reflect on the progress and achievements of the last half century and consider the future of linked data in Australia. This paper outlines Australia's data linkage journey, from its beginning in the 1970s up to the present day. Current challenges and plans for future development are also discussed.

2. The Early Years: Ad Hoc and Other Linkages (1970–1994)

In 1967, Professor Michael Hobbs returned to Western Australia from Oxford University, where he had been involved with the Oxford Record Linkage Study [5]. In 1970, he published a plan for the introduction of medical record linkage studies in Australia [1]. The plan included the initial linkage of birth, marriage and death records, census data, perinatal mortality and hospital morbidity records. This could be subsequently supplemented by:

"Records of physical or mental disability
Records of exposure to new industrial processes
Prescriptions of selected drugs
Notifications of infectious disease." [1]

Additional elements of the plan were described as follows:

"A plan for the introduction of medical record linkage studies in Australia on a National or State-wide basis must therefore include the following:

1. The interest and co-operation of the Bureau of Census and Statistics.
2. Preferably the introduction of a unique numbering system, but failing this, the collection of uniform identifying data on all records for which linkage is planned, either routinely or on an ad hoc basis.
3. The agreement by holders of important data to the release of information for linkage procedures under the auspices of the Bureau of Census and Statistics.
4. The realization by users of such data that tabulations identifying individual persons will not be practicable.
5. The awakening of interest in, and realization of the uses of, record linkage in Government Departments, Medical Administrators and research workers.
6. The implementation of a pilot record linkage scheme in Western Australia." [1]

This plan was the beginning of an Australian national linkage system which 51 years later incorporates many elements of the original plan. However, in 1970, systematic approaches to data linkage at the state or national level were still a long way off. Professor Hobbs and three other Western Australian researchers, Professor Bruce Armstrong, Professor Fiona Stanley and Professor D'Arcy Holman, were instrumental over the next 25 years in achieving a systematic data linkage system in Western Australia [1,5–7].

Western Australia was well positioned to have a population-based data linkage system as it was the only state to have implemented a state-wide hospital reporting system. From the mid-1970s, this included the standardised collection of names, which enabled high-quality linkage. Other elements that proved essential to the establishment of the Western Australian Data Linkage System were researcher champions including Professors Hobbs, Stanley and Holman, who understood the value of linked data, had the persistence to obtain it and the skills to use it, as well as strong collaboration between the Western Australian Department of Health and the University of Western Australia [6].

In 1977, Professor Stanley's research group established the Western Australian Maternal and Child Health Research Database, which was later housed at the Institute for Child

Health Research (now Telethon Kids Institute). This was a linked database containing the following state-wide data collections:

- Midwives notifications,
- Birth records,
- Death records,
- Hospital morbidity,
- The WA Birth Defects Registry (now the WA Register of Developmental Anomalies), and
- The Cerebral Palsy Register.

This unique linked data collection was an extremely valuable resource for a wide range of maternal and child health research, particularly the causes of stillbirth and risks factors for cerebral palsy [8]. The types of research supported included:

- Descriptive epidemiology of perinatal and paediatric outcomes [9],
- Case control studies [10],
- Cohort studies [11], and
- Studies to evaluate care [12].

During this time, Professors Stanley and Bower conducted their world leading research on the link between folate deficiency and neural tube defects [13]. Later, they went on to demonstrate that folate supplementation and fortification prevent these defects, a major contribution to public health [14].

3. The Introduction of State-Based Systematic Data Linkage: The Western Australian Data Linkage Branch and New South Wales Centre for Health Record Linkage (1995–2008)

3.1. Establishment and Development of the Western Australian Data Linkage Branch

In 1994–1995, Professor Holman was appointed as the inaugural Chair in Public Health at the University of Western Australia. Professors Holman, Hobbs and others put in a successful application to the Western Australian Lotteries Commission to establish a Health Services Research Linked Database [5]. The three-year grant enabled establishment of a data linkage unit within the Western Australian Department of Health. The initiative was supported by Professor Ian Rouse, the Department of Health's Director of Health Statistics and Dr John Bass was the first linker. Initial work was focused on creating probabilistic linkages within and between six core data collections, including births, deaths, hospital separations, midwives notification and cancer registry data [15,16].

The Lotteries Commission grant concluded in 1997–1998 and Dr Merran Smith, the then Director of the Department of Health's Heath Information Centre, submitted a successful proposal to establish data linkage as a core Departmental service. Additional health data collections were added to the data linkage system and additional staff were taken on to meet the growing demand for linked data. In 1999, the Department of Health became the principal funder and the Western Australian Data Linkage Branch which incorporated the data linkage unit was established within the Health Information Centre. The Western Australian Data Linkage System was one of only five such comprehensive systems in the world at the time [16]. Further information about the Western Australian Data Linkage Branch is available at https://www.datalinkage-wa.org.au/ (accessed on 21 October 2021).

A Management Committee was subsequently established to oversee the Western Australian linked data resources. This included representatives of the Department of Health, the University of Western Australia and the Institute for Child Health Research.

In 2002, an initiative commenced to create intergenerational family linkages (the Family Connections project) [17]. Data from other Western Australian Government agencies was also incorporated into the Western Australian Data Linkage System, including data from Education, Community Services and Justice Departments. Some data from these agencies was subsequently housed in a Custodian Controlled Research Extracts Server (CARES) to facilitate supply of linked data for approved projects [18].

3.2. Establishment of the Centre for Health Record Linkage (CHeReL)

In 1994, the then New South Wales Department of Health established a record linkage service to support health research and management of health services. In 2005, following marked increases in the demand for linked data, the Sax Institute commissioned Professor Holman and others from Western Australia to develop a case for a data linkage facility in New South Wales and to recommend a preferred model based on international best practice and stakeholders views. In 2006, eight organisations including New South Wales Health, the Australian Capital Territory Department of Health, Cancer Institute New South Wales and the Sax Institute, agreed to contribute funding for the first three years of operation of the CHeReL. The CHeReL subsequently transitioned to a business unit of New South Wales Health, primarily funded by the New South Wales Ministry of Health. It is of note that the CHeReL was established to undertake data linkage for both New South Wales and the Australian Capital Territory and this arrangement is continuing [19]. Further information about the CHeReL is available at https://www.cherel.org.au/ (accessed on 21 October 2021).

3.3. Challenges and Benefits

Challenges to establishing the Western Australian and New South Wales/Australian Capital Territory data linkage systems included support from decision-makers to establish the systems. For both the Western Australian Data Linkage System and the CHeReL, support from research users was a significant factor with each starting out as a collaboration between research groups and government agencies. It is of note that both units moved to a majority government agency support within a few years of establishment and both are now located within their respective state government health agency.

The Western Australia and New South Wales/Australian Capital Territory initiatives demonstrated the benefit of routinely updated, population-based, data linkage systems rather than ad hoc, project-based data linkages. Once established, there were many other benefits including cheaper projects, better data and improved privacy protection [15]. However, the time needed to obtain project approvals was often lengthy, especially for complex projects, and there were delays in supply of linked data. There were also challenges with linkage of data between Australian jurisdictions.

Privacy and confidentiality concerns from data custodians and the community were always a high priority and shaped the approach to systematic linkage in Western Australia and New South Wales. The use of the "best practice protocol", which requires the separation of identifiers from health data as well as the separation of roles, i.e., the people with access to the identifiers do not have access to the health data, was central to addressing these concerns [20].

In addition, strong community support for data linkage activities is essential to running a successful data linkage system. Both these data linkage systems have incorporated community involvement activities in their development and operations. In Western Australia, the Consumer and Community Health Research Network established in 1998 by the School of Population Health at the University of Western Australia has been particularly influential and supportive [21].

Moral and ethical issues around balancing all the interests at play, not just privacy, also had to be tackled. These issues included the protection of government interests and the possibility that not using linked data could result in harms by preventing or delaying health and health service improvements [22–24].

3.4. Early Cross-Jurisdictional Linkage

Australia is a federation with a complex health system. The Australian Government is responsible for some aspects of this system, with state and territory governments responsible for other aspects. As a result, some population health data is held by Australian Government agencies while other data is separately held by government agencies in six states and two territories.

One of the first examples of cross-jurisdiction data linkage in Australia was the Australian Cancer Statistics Clearing House. This was established in 1986 at the Australian Institute of Health and Welfare (AIHW). It linked cancer registry and death data from cancer registries in Australian states and territories to provide national cancer information. However, this data was not routinely linked to other population health data.

In 1998, discussions commenced to enable linkage of Australian Government Medical Benefits Schedule (MBS) payments and Pharmaceutical Benefits Scheme (PBS) data to the Western Australian linked hospitalisations and death data for a project on diabetes. A Memorandum of Understanding (MoU) to cover the linkage was developed between the (then) Commonwealth Department of Health and Aged Care, the Health Department of Western Australia, the University of Western Australia, the AIHW and the Health Insurance Commission. The MoU was signed in 2001 with particular support from the Secretary of Commonwealth Health (Mr Andrew Podger), the Commissioner of the Health Department of Western Australian (Mr Alan Bansemer) and the Director of AIHW (Dr Richard Madden) and the linkages were undertaken [20]. In 2003, the arrangement was expanded to establish a population-based, cross-jurisdiction linked data resource. The arrangement was supported by a cross-jurisdiction management committee which also considered applications for access to the linked data. It was the first time that this type of population-based, cross-jurisdiction data linkage resource was available in Australia. It enabled important research projects on topics such as potentially inappropriate medications in the elderly and the impact of regular primary care on outcomes of people with chronic diseases to be completed [25–28].

3.5. Challenges and Achievements

Challenges in establishing and accessing the cross-jurisdiction linked data resource included complex legal frameworks, lengthy project approval processes and delays in data supply. Changes in personnel in participating agencies also had an impact, with new appointees not always as supportive of cross-jurisdiction data linkage as their predecessors. The resource was last updated in 2007 and subsequently discontinued. Each of the challenges identified through the cross-jurisdiction data linkage project was complex in its own right and none was amenable to a simple solution. These challenges informed plans for the development of a more coordinated Australian data linkage system (see Section 4 below).

Although the resource was discontinued, the work clearly demonstrated the feasibility of population-based linkage of Australian Government and state government data, at both the governance and technical levels. It also highlighted the importance of access to cross-jurisdiction linked data in the Australian context.

4. National and Cross-Jurisdictional Data Linkage: The Population Health Research Network (PHRN) (2009–2021)

4.1. Establishment of the PHRN

In its 2004–05 Budget, the Australian Government announced the implementation of the National Collaborative Research Infrastructure Strategy (NCRIS) with the objective of bringing more strategic direction to the investment in national research infrastructure. This was followed in 2006 by the first NCRIS Strategic Roadmap. The Roadmap was developed after extensive national consultation and set the priorities for the Australian Government's investment in national research infrastructure.

The 2006 Roadmap proposed the scoping of a coordinated national data linkage capability.

"One possibility is that the capability could be modelled on the system that is being implemented in Western Australia . . . . A national system might comprise a network of such data linkage units with oversight by a coordination authority provided with both funding and staff capable of providing both intellectual leadership and administrative support" [29].

A lengthy national scoping and consultation period followed, with the final investment plan for a national data linkage capability accepted in 2009. The investment plan identified the University of Western Australia as lead agent for the PHRN and covered the establishment of a central coordinating office at the University, four new state/territory data linkage units based on the Western Australian model to complement the existing units in Western Australia and New South Wales, a national data linkage unit and a secure, remote access, data laboratory. The investment plan was designed to deal with the challenges of the complex Australian health system, to improve health and well-being, and enhance the effectiveness and efficiency of health services.

Contracts were signed and the establishment of PHRN commenced in April 2009 with the appointment of the Chief Executive. A detailed description of the PHRN data linkage infrastructure was published in 2019 [30]. Further information about PHRN is available at https://www.phrn.org.au/ (accessed on 21 October 2021).

Australia is a federation of six states and two self-governing territories which together make up the Commonwealth of Australia. State and territory governments are responsible for some aspects of health care, while the Australian Government is responsible for other aspects. The networked and coordinated approach to a national data linkage system implemented by the PHRN is a response to the unique characteristics of the federation and the Australian health system. This approach has similarities to the Health Data Research Network Canada which is working towards harmonizing data and linkage systems across many provinces [31]. Other smaller single jurisdiction nations such as New Zealand and Denmark have implemented centralized linkage systems, an approach which was not feasible in Australia [32,33].

4.2. Challenges and Achievements

The establishment of a national, coordinated data linkage infrastructure across nine jurisdictions should not be underestimated. While a distributed, federated system was the agreed approach, it also posed a number of challenges including:

- Standardisation of data and metadata across jurisdictions;
- Standardisation or benchmarking of linkage methods;
- Standardising, harmonising or coordinating approval requirements and processes;
- Different legislation, regulation, policy and culture between jurisdictions;
- Varying levels of data linkage experience and expertise between jurisdictions.

Another challenge was to get all jurisdictions to participate. While a majority of jurisdictions participated from the outset, it is only since 2011 that all Australian jurisdictions have participated.

Being a truly national network that links data from all Australian, state and territory governments was a priority for the PHRN from the beginning. Achieving participation from all jurisdictions meant supporting a high level of flexibility in how the data linkage infrastructure was developed, implemented and operated in each jurisdiction. Strict requirements for each jurisdiction to implement and operate in specific nationally agreed ways would have delayed the participation of some jurisdictions and it is possible that a national network of any kind may not have been achieved. However, the distributed approach resulted in differences in data linked, linkage methods and approval processes across jurisdictions, which make multi- and cross-jurisdictional research projects more complex than they would be with a standardised national approach [34,35].

To help address these challenges, the PHRN holds regular meetings with senior officers in participating organisations and hosts regular forums for technical staff. It is also working with jurisdictions to establish enduring cross-jurisdiction data linkage and related linked data assets.

A further challenge has been Australia's complex authorising environment, with each jurisdiction having its own set of enabling legislation and related policies and practice. PHRN continues to participate in jurisdictional and national processes aimed at simplifying the authorising environment. One success was the establishment of mutual acceptance of ethical review for data linkage projects. The PHRN also established and continues to operate an Online Application System and related services to assist researcher access to cross-jurisdiction linked data. There is strong growth in demand for this service [36].

The PHRN's most significant achievement is the establishment of a coordinated national system of cross-jurisdiction linkage. This system is internationally unique and enables health and human services data from different jurisdictions about the same individual to be linked and accessed. All Australian jurisdictions now have at least 10 years of their core population health data linked. Over 210 data collections are routinely linked and there are more than 15 billion records in the national linkage system. There is also regular linkage to national clinical registries and large longitudinal cohorts. In addition, Australian linked data is being increasingly used for clinical trials. There has been a steady increase in the number of data applications and peer reviewed publications using linked data since the establishment of the PHRN [36–38].

PHRN also pioneered national secure remote access data laboratories in Australia. The first, the Secure Unified Research Environment at the Sax Institute in Sydney, is now a well-used environment trusted by custodians across Australia to provide access to sensitive unit record data [36,38].

Research using PHRN linked data has positively impacted many aspects of health and other human services across Australia. This includes changes to government policy as well as changes in clinical practice. Information on impacts is available on the PHRN website [39]. One important example relates to the introduction of Human Papilloma Virus (HPV) vaccination to prevent cervical cancer. The vaccine was introduced in Australia in 2007 and monitored by linking vaccine registers to cervical smear registers in two states (Queensland and Victoria) [40–42]. Findings from these and related studies resulted in a change to Australia's cervical cancer screening program, with cytology screening every two years replaced with more accurate HPV screening every five years. The current COVID-19 pandemic is a further example, with Australia's linked data playing a significant part in jurisdiction responses to the pandemic [43].

While there has been an expansion of population-based data linkage capability across the globe in recent years, Australia remains one of a relatively small number of countries with a national population-based data linkage capability.

5. The Future of Data Linkage in Australia

The demand for access to high-quality linked data from an ever-expanding range of sources (omics, environment, clinical records, wearable devices, social media, etc.) is likely to accelerate over coming years. This demand will come from a wide range of users including governments, academia and private industry.

Close collaboration will be required across Australian jurisdictions, the research sector and industry to meet this demand, including to source the data required, routinely link across jurisdictions and provide access to linked data in efficient and safe ways. Changes to Australia's very complex authorising environment may also be needed to ensure that the rights and interests of stakeholders are carefully considered and the approval and access processes are proportionate to the risks as systems evolve. New technical advances in computing infrastructure and analytical techniques will make data linkage and the analysis and management of linked data more accurate, efficient and safe. New approaches to metadata and data standardisation for huge volumes of data from very different sources will also be required to enable people to find suitable data, and plan and execute their research.

In addition, it will be necessary to ensure that the Australian community supports and trusts the data linkage system and that linked data is used in ways that demonstrate clear public benefit. The community will need to become more data literate and better understand both the benefits that linked data can bring and the risks to individuals and groups. It may not be possible to ensure anonymity given the volume of data on each individual and the emerging analytical tools. A multi-pronged approach to community education and involvement will be required including:

- The provision of information about the benefits, risks and risk mitigation strategies on a range of communication platforms,
- Community involvement in setting the research agenda, and
- Community representation on decision making and advisory groups.

6. Conclusions

The first 50 years of data linkage development in Australia has provided a firm foundation for further expansion and development, and will help to ensure that Australia's linked health and human services data continues to be available to address the evolving challenges of the next half century.

Author Contributions: M.S. and F.F. both contributed equally to the article conception, literature review and drafting. All authors have read and agreed to the published version of the manuscript.

Funding: Merran Smith and Felicity Flack are employed by the University of Western Australia with funding from the Australian Government's National Collaborative Research Infrastructure Strategy via the Population Health Research Network.

Institutional Review Board Statement: Not applicable.

Informed Consent Statement: Not applicable.

Data Availability Statement: Not applicable.

Conflicts of Interest: Merran Smith and Felicity Flack are employed by the University of Western Australia with funding from the Australian Government's National Collaborative Research Infrastructure Strategy via the Population Health Research Network.

References

1. Hobbs, M.; McCall, M. Health statistics and record linkage in Australia. *J. Chronic Dis.* **1970**, *23*, 375–381. [CrossRef]
2. Machado, C.J.; Hill, K. Probabilistic record linkage and an automated procedure to minimize the undecided-matched pair problem. *Cad Saude Publica* **2004**, *20*, 915–925. [CrossRef] [PubMed]
3. Dunn, H.L. Record linkage. *Am. J. Public Health* **1946**, *36*, 1412–1416. [CrossRef]
4. Adams, C.; Flack, F.; Allen, J. Research using linked data. In *Sharing Linked Data for Health Research: Toward Better Decision Making*; Cambridge University Press: Cambridge, UK, in press.
5. Hobbs, M. Michael Hobbs Interview 24 January 2013. Available online: https://oralhistories.arts.uwa.edu.au/items/show/45 (accessed on 16 August 2021).
6. Armstrong, B.K.; Kricker, A. Record linkage—A vision renewed. *Aust. N. Z. J. Public Health* **1999**, *23*, 451–452. [CrossRef] [PubMed]
7. The School of Population Health Welcomes the Return of Professor Bruce Armstrong as Adjunct Professor. Available online: https://www.news.uwa.edu.au/archive/201512228287/appointments/school-population-health-welcomes-return-professor-bruce-armstrong-adjunct/ (accessed on 21 October 2021).
8. Stanley, F.J.; Croft, M.L.; Gibbins, J.; Read, A.W. A population database for maternal and child health research in Western Australia using record linkage. *Paediatr. Perinat. Epidemiol.* **1994**, *8*, 433–447. [CrossRef]
9. Stanley, F.J.; Hobbs, M.S. Perinatal outcome in Western Australia, 1968 to 1975 3. Causes of stillbirths and neonatal deaths excluding congenital malformations. *Med. J. Aust.* **1981**, *1*, 483–486. [CrossRef] [PubMed]
10. Alessandri, L.M.; Stanley, F.J.; Garner, J.B.; Newnham, J.; Walters, B.N.J. A case-control study of unexplained antepartum stillbirths. *BJOG Int. J. Obstet. Gynaecol.* **1992**, *99*, 711–718. [CrossRef] [PubMed]
11. Stanley, F.J.; English, D.R. Prevalence of and risk factors for cerebral palsy in a total population cohort of low-birthweight (less than 2000g) infants. *Dev. Med. Child Neurol.* **1986**, *28*, 559–568. [CrossRef] [PubMed]
12. Stanley, F.J.; Hobbs, M.S.T. Neonatal mortality and cerebral palsy: The impact of neonatal intensive care. *J. Paediatr. Child Health* **1980**, *16*, 35–39. [CrossRef]
13. Bower, C.; Stanley, F.J. Dietary folate as a risk factor for neural-tube defects: Evidence from a case-control study in Western Australia. *Med. J. Aust.* **1989**, *150*, 613–619. [CrossRef] [PubMed]
14. Bower, C.; Ryan, A.; Rudy, E.; Miller, M. Trends in neural tube defects in Western Australia. *Aust. N. Z. J. Public Health* **2002**, *26*, 150–151. [CrossRef] [PubMed]

15. Holman, C.D.; Bass, A.J.; Rosman, D.L.; Smith, M.B.; Semmens, J.B.; Glasson, E.J.; Brook, E.L.; Trutwein, B.; Rouse, I.L.; Watson, C.R.; et al. A decade of data linkage in Western Australia: Strategic design, applications and benefits of the WA data linkage system. *Aust. Health Rev.* **2008**, *32*, 766–777. [CrossRef] [PubMed]
16. Holman, C.D. *20 Years of Discovery and Advance 1994–5 to 2013–14*; University of Western Australia: Perth, Australia, 2014.
17. Glasson, E.J.; de Klerk, N.H.; Bass, A.J.; Rosman, D.L.; Palmer, L.J.; Holman, C.D.J. Cohort profile: The Western Australian family connections genealogical project. *Int. J. Epidemiol.* **2008**, *37*, 30–35. [CrossRef] [PubMed]
18. Eitelhuber, T.; Davis, G.; Rosman, D.L.; Glauert, R. Western Australia unveils advances in linked data delivery systems. *Aust. N. Z. J. Public Health* **2014**, *38*, 397–398. [CrossRef] [PubMed]
19. Irvine, K.; Hall, R.; Taylor, L. Centre for Health Record Linkage: Expanding access to linked population data for NSW and the ACT, Australia. *Int. J. Popul. Data Sci.* **2019**, *4*. [CrossRef]
20. Kelman, C.; Bass, A.; Holman, C. Research use of linked health data-a best practice protocol. *Aust. N. Z. J. Public Health* **2002**, *26*, 251–255. [CrossRef]
21. Consumer and Community Involvement Program. About Us. Available online: https://cciprogram.org/about-us/ (accessed on 23 August 2021).
22. Yazahmeidi, B.; Holman, C.D.J. A survey of suppression of public health information by Australian governments. *Aust. N. Z. J. Public Health* **2007**, *31*, 551–557. [CrossRef]
23. McKenzie, A.; Wale, J.; McLure, K.; Hill, I.; Rumley, H.; Colbung, M.; Daniels, B.; Powell, L.; Cuesta-Briand, B. Response to 'A survey of suppression of public health information by Australian governments'. *Public Health* **2008**, *32*, 90–91. [CrossRef] [PubMed]
24. Allen, J.; Holman, C.D.; Meslin, E.M.; Stanley, F. Privacy protectionism and health information: Is there any redress for harms to health? *J. Law Med.* **2013**, *21*, 473–485.
25. Price, S.D.; Holman, C.D.; Sanfilippo, F.M.; Emery, J.D. Are older Western Australians exposed to potentially inappropriate medications according to the Beers criteria? A 13-year prevalence study. *Australas J. Ageing* **2014**, *33*, E39–E48. [CrossRef]
26. Price, S.D.; Holman, C.D.; Sanfilippo, F.M.; Emery, J.D. Association between potentially inappropriate medications from the Beers criteria and the risk of unplanned hospitalization in elderly patients. *Ann. Pharmacother.* **2014**, *48*, 6–16. [CrossRef] [PubMed]
27. Einarsdóttir, K.; Preen, D.B.; Emery, J.D.; Holman, C.D. Regular primary care decreases the likelihood of mortality in older people with epilepsy. *Med. Care* **2010**, *48*, 472–476. [CrossRef] [PubMed]
28. Einarsdóttir, K.; Preen, D.B.; Emery, J.D.; Kelman, C.; Holman, C.D. Regular primary care lowers hospitalisation risk and mortality in seniors with chronic respiratory diseases. *J. Gen. Intern. Med.* **2010**, *25*, 766–773. [CrossRef] [PubMed]
29. National Collaborative Research Infrastructure Strategy Strategic Roadmap. 2006. Available online: https://www.dese.gov.au/national-research-infrastructure/resources/national-collaborative-research-infrastructure-strategy-strategic-roadmap-2006 (accessed on 13 September 2021).
30. Flack, F.; Smith, M. The Population Health Research Network—Population data centre profile. *Int. J. Pop. Data Sci.* **2019**, *4*, 1130. [CrossRef]
31. About Health Data Research Network Canada. Available online: https://www.hdrn.ca/en/about (accessed on 21 October 2021).
32. Integrated Data Infrastructure. Available online: https://www.stats.govt.nz/integrated-data/integrated-data-infrastructure/ (accessed on 21 October 2021).
33. The National Patient Register. Available online: https://econ.au.dk/the-national-centre-for-register-based-research/danish-registers/the-national-patient-register/ (accessed on 21 October 2021).
34. Productivity Commission 2017. Data Availability and Use: Overview & Recommendations, Report No. 82, Canberra. Available online: https://www.pc.gov.au/inquiries/completed/data-access/report (accessed on 28 October 2021).
35. Moore, H.C.; Guiver, T.; Woollacott, A.; De Klerk, N.; Gidding, H.F. Establishing a process for conducting cross-jurisdictional record linkage in Australia. *Aust. N. Z. J. Public Health* **2016**, *40*, 159–164. [CrossRef]
36. PHRN Annual Review 2019–20. Available online: https://www.phrn.org.au/media/82004/phrn-annual-review-2019-2020_digital-v10.pdf (accessed on 21 October 2021).
37. Young, A.; Flack, F. Recent trends in the use of linked data in Australia. *Aust. Health Rev.* **2018**, *42*, 584–590. [CrossRef]
38. SURE. Available online: https://www.saxinstitute.org.au/our-work/sure/ (accessed on 21 October 2021).
39. Impact Stories. Available online: https://www.phrn.org.au/for-the-community/impact-stories (accessed on 2 September 2021).
40. Brotherton, J.M.L.; Malloy, M.; Budd, A.C.; Saville, M.; Drennan, K.T.; Gertig, D.M. Effectiveness of less than three doses of quadrivalent human Papillomavirus vaccine against cervical intraepithelial neoplasia when administered using a standard dose spacing schedule: Observational cohort of young women in Australia. *Papillomavirus Res.* **2015**, *1*, 59–73. [CrossRef]
41. Clothier, H.J.; Lee, K.J.; Sundararajan, V.; Buttery, J.P.; Crawford, N.W. Human Papillomavirus vaccine in boys: Background rates of potential adverse events. *Med. J. Aust.* **2013**, *198*, 554–558. [CrossRef]
42. Crowe, E.; Pandeya, N.; Brotherton, J.M.L.; Dobson, A.J.; Kisely, S.; Lambert, S.B.; Whiteman, D.C. Effectiveness of quadrivalent human Papillomavirus vaccine for the prevention of cervical abnormalities: Case-control study nested within a population based screening programme in Australia. *Br. Med. J.* **2014**, *348*, g1458. [CrossRef]
43. Population Health Research Network. Linked Data in the Fight against COVID-19. Available online: https://www.phrn.org.au/media/82108/impact-story-linked-data-in-the-fight-against-covid-19.pdf (accessed on 23 August 2021).

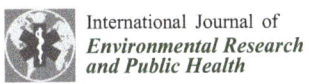

Communication

Using Data Integration to Improve Health and Welfare Insights

Linda R. Jensen

Australian Institute of Health and Welfare, 1 Thynne St., Bruce, ACT 2617, Australia; linda.jensen@aihw.gov.au

Abstract: The Australian Institute of Health and Welfare (AIHW) is a leader in the provision of high-quality health and welfare information. Its work program has built a strong evidence base for better decisions that deliver improved health and welfare outcomes. The evolution of the AIHW's data integration program has exemplified innovation in identifying and addressing key information gaps, as well as responsiveness to opportunities to develop and capture the data required to inform national priorities. The AIHW conducts data integration in partnership with data custodians and specialists in integration and analysis. A linkage project requiring the integration of Australian government data must be undertaken by an accredited integrating authority. The AIHW has met stringent criteria covering project governance, capability, and data management to gain this accreditation. In this capacity, the AIHW is trusted to integrate Australian government data for high-risk research projects. To date, the AIHW's integration projects have generated improved research outcomes that have identified vulnerable population groups, improved the understanding of health risk factors, and contributed to the development of targeted interventions. These projects have fostered new insights into dementia, disability, health service use, patient experiences of healthcare, and suicide. Upcoming projects aim to further the understanding of interrelationships between determinants of wellbeing.

Keywords: continuity of care; data; disability; dementia; health; health service use; integration; last year of life; linkage; suicide; veterans; welfare; wellbeing

Citation: Jensen, L.R. Using Data Integration to Improve Health and Welfare Insights. *Int. J. Environ. Res. Public Health* **2022**, *19*, 836. https://doi.org/10.3390/ijerph19020836

Academic Editors: Richard Madden and Jeanine M. Buchanich

Received: 1 November 2021
Accepted: 5 January 2022
Published: 12 January 2022

Publisher's Note: MDPI stays neutral with regard to jurisdictional claims in published maps and institutional affiliations.

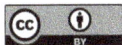

Copyright: © 2022 by the author. Licensee MDPI, Basel, Switzerland. This article is an open access article distributed under the terms and conditions of the Creative Commons Attribution (CC BY) license (https://creativecommons.org/licenses/by/4.0/).

1. Introduction

The Australian Institute of Health and Welfare (AIHW) is a leader in health and welfare information. Its analytical work program offers insights into how Australians interact with the health and welfare systems, through the analysis of a broad range of data sourced from surveys, administrative records, and service delivery functions. The outputs of the AIHW work program provide strong evidence as a basis for better policy and program delivery decisions that ultimately lead to improved health and welfare outcomes for Australians [1].

The AIHW is an international leader in data integration and has gained accreditation as an integrating authority [2,3]. This accreditation allows the AIHW to integrate Australian government data for statistical and research purposes.

In this context, the AIHW has developed an extensive data integration program that has provided opportunities to build richer analytical datasets, which can deliver research outcomes beyond what is possible from analysis of single data sources. The program of work has provided opportunities for the following:

- Broader level reporting and analysis—e.g., whole-population and national data;
- Addressing key data gaps by connecting content datasets that relate to a single entity;
- Analysis and reporting of rare or sensitive issues and events;
- Analysis of pathways taken through health and welfare systems and to understand the experience over a person's life course;
- Identification of specific population groups in broader administrative datasets—e.g., migrants or veterans.

The AIHW adheres to all relevant legislation and guidelines to ensure it upholds strict privacy and confidentiality requirements.

The AIHW seeks opportunities to drive innovation in the collection, use, and analysis of health and welfare information, to learn from international experience, and to develop approaches that align with best practice. The AIHW's international engagement includes the following:

- Participation in Organization for Economic Co-operation and Development (OECD) activities, including the Working Party on Health Statistics;
- Longstanding involvement with the World Health Organization, through the WHO Family of International Classifications Network (WHO-FIC), and as the designated Australian Collaborating Center (ACC) for the WHO-FIC;
- Collaboration with the Canadian Institute for Health Information, through sharing and comparing approaches, and participating in secondments across the agencies;
- Membership with the National Initiative Network, a collective that shares experiences in developing stronger frameworks to promote secondary use of health and wellbeing data;
- Partnership with The Five Eyes research collective, with a particular focus on international comparisons of data about veterans;
- Contact with the United States of America National Center for Health Statistics, Statistics New Zealand, and the Commonwealth Fund.

2. AIHW Data Integration Projects

To date, data integration projects undertaken by the AIHW have generated improved research outcomes for a number of specific population groups and health and welfare topics. This has supported the identification of vulnerable population groups, provided a better understanding of health and welfare risk factors, and contributed to the development of targeted interventions. The AIHW has addressed significant data gaps, extended analysis of complex relationships in health and welfare, and undertaken pioneering research that provides new insights into how Australians interact with health and welfare systems.

Projects are currently underway which seek to maximize the use of broad, national data assets to build a more holistic understanding of the interrelationships between the determinants of health and wellbeing for Australians. Some of these assets are held and maintained by the AIHW, while others are accessed in partnership with other Australian government agencies.

All AIHW data integration projects are conducted in partnership with a range of data custodians and specialists in data integration and analysis. Recent and upcoming AIHW data integration projects are described below.

2.1. Dementia

Dementia is a condition that is not consistently captured in individual datasets and is generally poorly captured in nationally representative surveys. The AIHW's capacity to monitor and report on dementia has been transformed through data integration, which has enabled the following key achievements:

- Better identification of people with dementia in Australia, leading to better coverage in reporting and more accurate understanding of disease prevalence, comorbidities, risk factors, and population groups with dementia.
- Developing an understanding of the course of disease over time for people with records of dementia including the potential to examine factors that affect the use of health and aged care services. Records of dementia may include a specific diagnosis, or recorded use of dementia-specific medications for diagnosis by proxy.
- Understanding the consequences of dementia diagnoses in many more aspects of a person's life than previously reportable—e.g., on work and income, or receipt of welfare or disability support payments.

Data integration has also extended the use of existing data. For example, the AIHW has developed models that identify predictors of early dementia in a dataset that contains no dementia diagnosis information [4]. Ultimately, this information can be used to more accurately estimate dementia incidence and prevalence, as well as contribute to filling information gaps in the primary and specialist care domains.

The AIHW's dementia data integration projects are providing new and important information on people with dementia in Australia, making use of data from the five-yearly Australian Census of Population and Housing, plus welfare data that would previously have been of little use for studies of dementia without data integration.

2.2. Disability

The AIHW is working in partnership with national and state-level governments to integrate government data to develop a National Disability Data Asset (NDDA). This project brings together deidentified data from over 50 datasets, sourced from all levels of government, to build a linked administrative data asset that can support reporting under the outcomes framework of a new National Disability Strategy (NDS).

The NDDA is currently in its pilot phase, which is focused on developing processes for sharing data among government data custodians, to gain a better understanding of people's life experiences. Analyses of five public policy topics are being used to demonstrate the potential of using linked data, as well as to inform design for a potential enduring asset. These topics include early childhood support, experiences with the justice system, pathways from education to employment, and services and support for people with disability and mental health issues. The pilot phase aims to derive a comprehensive measure of disability and demonstrate how linked administrative data can support an outcomes framework under the NDS.

This pilot builds on AIHW's health and welfare data expertise, which has supported NDDA delivery partners to develop and capture previously unavailable information on people with disability. The complexity of negotiating ethical approval, navigating Australian government legislation requirements, and ensuring privacy compliance of personal information has proven challenging. As the integrating authority for the pilot phase of the NDDA, the AIHW has established rigorous end-to-end data governance and management arrangements in accordance with privacy, legal, and technical aspects of the supply, to ensure that data of value can safely be included in the asset. A key achievement is the collaboration among the AIHW, the Australian Bureau of Statistics (ABS), and state government partners to create the pilot dataset.

Early learnings from the pilot include the potential to improve data sharing arrangements by streamlining governance and leveraging existing data integration infrastructure at a national level. A system that facilitates delivery of timely and relevant data will inform national priorities and support improved policy development, program design, and service delivery for people with disability.

Research findings on the five topic areas will be available in late 2021. Learnings from the pilot will inform options for an enduring data asset beyond 2021, including priority data for inclusion, data integration models, approved uses of the NDDA, and appropriate governance models for the asset.

2.3. Health Service Use: Last Year of Life

The AIHW is using the National Integrated Health Services Information (NIHSI) integrated data asset to examine health service use patterns and their corresponding costs for Australians who lived their last year of life between 2011–2012 and 2016–2017. The project aims to identify key factors related to the variability in the patterns of health service use in the last year of life. The key factors may include patient characteristics of age, sex, remoteness, socioeconomic group, and cause of death. Comparisons will be made to the health service use of the rest of the population (those who did not die) with otherwise similar characteristics.

Key analysis datasets used in this project are the National Death Index (NDI) linked to data on health service use, pharmaceutical prescriptions, and hospital, emergency department, and residential aged care.

Results from this analysis will provide information on Australians' interaction with a range of health services prior to death. They will help to identify the characteristics of Australians who are not accessing the services they need in their last year of life. This will provide useful information for healthcare professionals and policymakers.

Analyses for both service utilization and costs are underway, with an interactive web report planned for release in late 2021.

2.4. Patient Experiences of Continuity of Care

The AIHW developed the Coordination of Healthcare (CHC) study in partnership with the ABS to fill an important data gap and provide information on patients' experiences of continuity of care across Australia [5]. The study, which included people aged 45 and over, used a survey and data integration to examine patient experiences of continuity of care across Australia and importantly by the Primary Health Network [6]. The survey collected self-reported experiences of health service use including general practitioners (GPs), specialists, hospitals, and emergency departments. It also asked about health status including long-term health conditions, medication use, and sociodemographic characteristics.

Responses from consenting participants were linked to their administrative health data, including health service use and pharmaceutical prescription data, plus hospital and emergency department data for the pre- and post-survey period. The resulting integrated dataset provides a unique source of information on patient experiences, health status, and service use data [7]. This data linkage has enabled researchers to quantify and describe the actual use of health services (such as GP and hospital visits) and compare it with self-reported data on people's experiences of healthcare.

2.5. Suicide

The AIHW has used data from the Multi Agency Data Integration Project (MADIP) national data asset to analyze the contribution of different social determinants to death by suicide in Australia. The results will inform future policy development to help prevent deaths by suicide.

The 2011 Australian Census of Population and Housing was linked to the ABS Death Registrations collection to form the analysis population, which was then linked to key analysis datasets, covering a range of health and welfare topics. The quality of income data from MADIP was improved using a synthetic measure developed by the Australian National University, based on taxation and social security payment data. Application of a weighting methodology addressed issues with linkage coverage.

Initial analyses on cumulative risks of dying from suicide by educational attainment and employment status were released publicly [8].

Multiple statistical models have been developed (including a competing risk model) to provide a better understanding of the contribution of different social determinants—sex, age, indigenous status, occupation, marital status, household composition, and personal income—to deaths by suicide. Preliminary results, intended for publication in September 2021, provide useful insights into associations between certain social determinants and the risk of suicide.

2.6. Veterans

Because of their unique service experience, many permanent, reserve, and ex-serving Australian Defense Force (ADF) members ('veterans') and their families experience challenges beyond those typically experienced by the general Australian population [9,10].

In collaboration with the Australian national government's Departments of Defense and Veterans' Affairs, the AIHW is monitoring and reporting on the health and welfare status of veterans. Outcomes for veterans are compared to those of the broader Australian population, to identify specific risk and protective factors, as well as the social determinants of health and welfare of Australian veterans.

To date, specific analyses in this work program have focused on understanding the following:

- Overall causes of death and incidence of suicide for current serving and ex-serving ADF members [11];
- The welfare of ex-serving ADF members, from analysis of several topics including housing, social support, education and skills, employment, and income and finance;
- The use of healthcare services by ex-serving ADF members;
- Use of subsidized prescription medication by ex-serving ADF members;
- Health status, risk factors, and health conditions [12].

Under the veterans' analysis work program, the AIHW integrates ADF personnel data with other government datasets to enable identification of veterans in a range of administrative datasets including death registries, Pharmaceutical Benefits Scheme, and Homelessness Support Services. A key development resulting from this work program has been the addition of a veteran identifier flag to the MADIP, which will allow identification of veterans in the broad range of datasets included in MADIP, to inform on aspects such as employment, income, education, and social service use.

The analytical outputs of the veterans' analysis work program are building a profile of Australia's veterans which is helping to drive data improvement, inform development of policy and targeted interventions, and ultimately, improve the wellbeing of Australia's veterans [13].

3. The AIHW Data Integration Process

Australian government entities strongly support data integration, to maximize the benefits and use of government data assets and, importantly, to reduce the burden on individual respondents and data providers.

To protect privacy and confidentiality, as well as maximize the public benefit of its research, the AIHW integration program takes place in a secure and regulated environment. The AIHW integration environment is characterized by strict adherence to privacy principles through appropriate governance and approvals, strong strategic partnerships, secure data integration processes, and the creation and maintenance of high-quality data assets.

3.1. Governance and Approvals

The AIHW's data integration environment adheres to, and is bound by, both mandatory requirements and best practice policies and processes. These include Australian government legislation, policy, and guidelines, data security protocols, approval by ethics or human research ethics committees, data custodians and data access committees, and adherence to national and international best practice and frameworks including the *Privacy Act 1988* and the *Australian Privacy Principles (APPs)* [14,15]. The AIHW's data governance framework provides details of our strong data governance arrangements, including descriptions of key concepts, governance structures and roles, and the systems and tools that support them [16]. In addition, the AIHW's privacy policy outlines how the AIHW handles personal information [17].

The AIHW Ethics Committee is established under Section 16 of the *Australian Institute of Health and Welfare Act* [18]. Its functions and membership are prescribed in the *Australian Institute of Health and Welfare (Ethics Committee) Regulations 2018* [19]. All data linkage projects must be approved by the AIHW Ethics Committee and other relevant ethics committees where appropriate. The ethics application must include evidence of consultation with relevant stakeholders, including the general community, to establish their support and trust. Projects are required to be transparent and must make results publicly available. As part of this, information about projects and their outcomes are also published on the AIHW website.

All projects are assessed against the Five Safes, which is an internationally recognized approach to considering strategic, privacy, security, ethical, and operational risks as part of a holistic assessment of the risks associated with data sharing or release [20]. Guided

by this framework, the AIHW applies the following criteria to assess all new integration projects and assign a risk rating:
- Safe Projects—Is the use of the data appropriate (legal, moral, and ethical)?
- Safe Users—Can the users be trusted to use it in an appropriate manner?
- Safe Data—Is there a disclosure risk in releasing the data itself?
- Safe Settings—Does the access facility prevent unauthorized use?
- Safe Output—Are the statistical results non-disclosive [21]?

Output is governed by the *Australian Institute of Health and Welfare Act 1987*, and strict review of outputs by AIHW's data integration managers ensures protection of privacy and confidentiality [18].

3.2. Strategic Partnerships

Strong relationships with stakeholders are essential to the production of accurate information and to achieving improved data collection practices. The AIHW collaborates closely with experts in data integration and has effective data partnerships with government entities—national, state, and local, as well as with universities, research centers, nongovernment organizations, and other experts throughout the country. For current integration projects, the AIHW engages with government experts on health, education, community services, and housing.

The AIHW is working closely with the ABS, to develop a consistent national integration system. This partnership aims to maximize the use of existing survey, Australian Census of Population and Housing, and government administrative data. By supporting the use of consistent national data standards and approaches to collection, the AIHW and ABS can build and coordinate secure access to integrated national assets that support multiple analytical uses.

All data integration work is performed under guidance from a number of specialist advisory committees. In addition, the AIHW engages with consumers to continue to build community trust.

3.3. Quality Data

The AIHW collects, hosts, analyzes, and disseminates data that support the understanding of important health and welfare issues, and that are critical to good policymaking and effective service delivery.

The AIHW Quality Management Framework (QMF) is used to manage risk and maintain quality. The QMF draws on aspects of separate enterprise architecture, quality gate, data validation, and project management models developed by other national and international organizations. Application of the QMF across all stages of data integration and analysis projects maximizes the potential to deliver outputs that support and inform policy development and decision making.

The five key elements of the QMF are as follows:
- Statistical risk—Managing statistical risks, which can occur at all stages and levels in the statistical production cycle, is key to maintaining data quality. To minimize statistical risk, the QMF provides clear definitions of the risks to data quality, as well as their significance (major, medium or minor), and provides guidance on developing strategies for their management.
- Project management—All statistical projects must complete a risk assessment at the planning stage. The project brief lists major risks, and any risks already realized are elevated to issues. Strategies for mitigation and management must be included. The risk assessment feeds into the design of the quality assurance and data validation strategies for each project. Risks are reviewed regularly throughout the project's lifecycle.
- Quality assurance (QA)—QA strategies are particularly useful for identifying medium-level statistical risks and quality issues. They give a more detailed view of the factors impacting risks and data quality, often from a process perspective. The QMF provides context, generic tools, and a broad operational model to assist with the design of

consistent QA strategies. It uses a set of generic gates to improve the early detection of errors or flaws in production processes. It also defines the roles and responsibilities for managing quality and performance measures to facilitate quality gate assessments.
- Data validation—Data validation processes present the last opportunity to detect, resolve, and treat important errors before the data are released to clients. Validation also enables anomalous data that are correct to be identified and explained. The QMF provides templates, guidance, and explanatory notes to assist with data validation work.
- Reference models—The QMF is based on reference models that integrate critical project management activities into the statistical production process, provide guidance on quality assurance and data validation work, and define the roles and responsibilities of stakeholders across project phases. These models can also be used to benchmark, monitor, understand, and streamline production processes, improving responsiveness and capability into the future.

3.4. Data Integration

The AIHW provides a secure linkage environment for all approved linkage activity. The Data Integration Service Center (DISC) is a separate computer network that is not connected to the internet or any other AIHW system and includes strict protocols and procedures for physical security, data security, and manager review of outputs to ensure ethics compliance.

All AIHW data integration activities, regardless of risk level, are undertaken within the DISC. The linkage process is designed for each new project, around the following principles:
- The separation principle means that no one working with the data can view both the linking (identifying) information (such as name, address, date of birth) together with the merged analysis (content) data (such as clinical information, health service, or medication usage) in an integrated dataset. Under the separation principle, data integration is performed in three stages—separation, linkage, and merging. Each stage has a separate domain within the specific project in the DISC. Each domain is accessible only by staff holding the specified role, and staff members can only perform one role in each project.
- Linkage is done on datasets containing essential data items only,
- Sophisticated probabilistic data linkage methodology is used to achieve the best possible linkage results. The linkage is performed using linkage software developed by the AIHW.
- Output is appropriately confidentialized before it is made available to researchers, in accordance with appropriate legislation and the requirements of data custodians.

4. Opportunities and Challenges

Data integration has increased the capacity to fill key data gaps and support better decisions to develop and deliver targeted interventions to those who are at risk. By combining data from different sources, and harnessing expertise through strategic partnerships, the AIHW data integration program has provided opportunities for the following:
- Enhanced analysis—the research potential of integrated datasets is greater than of those based on a singular source. Integrated data have a broader coverage of topics and provide greater potential to examine interrelationships between topics.
- Cleaner data—the combination of data from different sources enables the development of improved data checks that can enhance the quality of the separate data sources. This can be achieved through the development of data collection standards or definitions of data items that relate to standard classifications.
- Cost effectiveness—linking data collected for other purposes is far cheaper than obtaining similar data through surveys and longitudinal studies. Reuse of existing administrative data greatly reduces the costs associated with both provision and collection.
- Improved coverage—linked datasets can represent a large sample, allowing broader-level reporting that is not possible from individual survey data. Use of integrated

data can assist to address issues associated with small numbers. This both protects the privacy of individuals and enhances analysis and reporting of sensitive or rare events.
- Identification of target groups—linking information about target groups, e.g., migrants or veterans, creates broader datasets that support the analysis of wellbeing and identification of risk factors for these groups, without the requirement to ask for this detailed information in administrative datasets.
- Longitudinal analysis—integrating datasets over time can allow the analysis of pathways through health and welfare systems or over the life course of an individual or cohort.

While offering many opportunities, the development of and access to a broad range of data assets for integration present many challenges such as the following:

- Coordination of the large and complex data integration landscape, involving data assets from all levels of government.
- Complex governance arrangements—including understanding the implications of relevant legislation, policies, and ethics. This requires a considerable amount of time and documentation.
- Managing liaison and approvals across multiple data custodians, especially across different levels of government. Integration projects drawing data from multiple sources typically require approvals from multiple ethics committees or custodians.
- Building community trust and engagement.
- Methodological challenges, where weighting practices may be required to ensure appropriate representativeness of the data.
- Data inconsistencies across input data sources. Data used in integration projects are often collected for service delivery or administrative purposes. They may have different definitions, concepts, specifications, coding, classifications, standards, and quality across sources.
- The need to quickly develop expertise in new and complex data models, as well as new approaches to analysis. As demand continues to grow for accessible and large-scale linked data assets such as the NIHSI and NDDA, the AIHW is responding to more complex, cross-sector research questions.

In many cases, the source data for AIHW integration projects have not been used in this way before. The AIHW has invested considerable effort to assess their suitability to inform policies and meet research objectives through data integration.

To meet these challenges, maintain strong leadership in data integration, and ensure the ongoing utility of Australian government data to meet research objectives and inform decision making, the AIHW data integration work program will continue to focus on the following:

- Forming new and strengthening existing partnerships across all levels of government, to promote access to and use of data assets, as well as sharing of expertise.
- Promoting processes to safely share data for integration in national data assets that allows richer, deeper analysis of populations of interest. An example of this is the addition of population flags to national data assets, as in the AIHW veterans' analysis work program.
- Continuous improvement and innovation in data collection practices, including opportunities to harmonize the way data on topics of interest are defined and collected.
- Supporting the development of governance frameworks that facilitate data integration involving data assets from all levels of government, while maintaining the privacy and confidentiality of data about individuals, as well as meeting the specific requirements of data custodians for access to and use of their data.

Funding: This research article received no external funding. Data integration projects undertaken at AIHW, such as the projects described in this article, are predominantly funded through the Australian Commonwealth Government.

Institutional Review Board Statement: Data integration projects undertaken at AIHW are subject to approval by the AIHW Ethics Committee which is recognised by the National Health and Medical Research Council (NHMRC) as a properly constituted Human Research Ethics Committee as outlined in the National Statement on Ethical Conduct in Human Research. The integration projects described in this article were approved by the AIHW Ethics Committee at various times.

Informed Consent Statement: The integration projects described in this article sought waivers of consent where applicable as part of the ethics submission and approval process.

Acknowledgments: The AIHW acknowledges the participation of Joanna Abbs, Naomi Cobcroft, Fleur de Crespigny, Louise Gates, Linda Jensen, Sarah Jones, Paul Lukong, Leanne Luong, Anne-Marie Rushby, Rebecca Sullivan, and Caitlin Szigetvari in writing and reviewing of the manuscript.

Conflicts of Interest: The authors declare no conflict of interest.

References

1. Australian Government: Australian Institute of Health and Welfare (AIHW). Available online: https://www.aihw.gov.au/about-us (accessed on 6 July 2021).
2. AIHW. Available online: https://www.aihw.gov.au/our-services/data-linkage/our-secure-linkage-environment (accessed on 6 July 2021).
3. Australian Government. Available online: https://toolkit.data.gov.au/Data_Integration_-_Accredited_Integrating_Authorities.html (accessed on 6 July 2021).
4. AIHW. Available online: https://www.aihw.gov.au/reports/dementia/predicting-early-dementia-using-medicare-claims/contents/summary (accessed on 30 October 2021).
5. AIHW. Available online: https://www.aihw.gov.au/reports-data/health-welfare-overview/health-care-quality-performance/coordination-of-health-care (accessed on 26 August 2021).
6. Australian Government: Department of Health. Primary Health Networks. Available online: https://www.health.gov.au/initiatives-and-programs/phn (accessed on 26 August 2021).
7. Coordination of Health Care for Patients Aged 45 and Over by Primary Health Networks, Summary—Australian Institute of Health and Welfare. Available online: aihw.gov.au (accessed on 26 August 2021).
8. AIHW. Available online: https://www.aihw.gov.au/suicide-self-harm-monitoring/data/behaviours-risk-factors/social-factors-suicide (accessed on 26 August 2021).
9. AIHW. Available online: https://www.aihw.gov.au/reports-data/population-groups/veterans/overview (accessed on 6 July 2021).
10. AIHW. Available online: https://www.aihw.gov.au/reports/veterans/a-profile-of-australias-veterans-2018/summary (accessed on 6 July 2021).
11. AIHW. Available online: https://www.aihw.gov.au/reports/veterans/serving-and-ex-serving-adf-suicide-monitoring-2021 (accessed on 30 October 2021).
12. AIHW. Available online: https://www.aihw.gov.au/reports-data/population-groups/veterans/reports (accessed on 6 July 2021).
13. AIHW. Available online: https://www.aihw.gov.au/reports/veterans/adf-members-population-characteristics-2019 (accessed on 30 October 2021).
14. Australian Government. Available online: https://www.legislation.gov.au/Details/C2020C00237 (accessed on 19 August 2021).
15. Australian Government: Office of the Australian Information Commissioner. Available online: https://www.oaic.gov.au/privacy/australian-privacy-principles (accessed on 19 August 2021).
16. AIHW. Available online: https://www.aihw.gov.au/about-our-data/data-governance (accessed on 19 August 2021).
17. AIHW. Available online: https://www.aihw.gov.au/about-us/privacy-policy/aihw-privacy-policy (accessed on 30 August 2021).
18. Australian Government. Available online: https://www.legislation.gov.au/Series/C2004A03450 (accessed on 26 August 2021).
19. AIHW. Available online: https://www.legislation.gov.au/Details/F2018L00317 (accessed on 30 August 2021).
20. Five Safes. Available online: www.fivesafes.org (accessed on 6 July 2021).
21. AIHW. Available online: https://www.aihw.gov.au/about-our-data/data-governance/the-five-safes-framework (accessed on 6 July 2021).

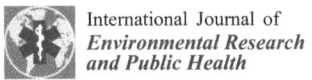

Review

Generating Real-World Evidence on the Quality Use, Benefits and Safety of Medicines in Australia: History, Challenges and a Roadmap for the Future

Sallie-Anne Pearson [1,*], Nicole Pratt [2], Juliana de Oliveira Costa [1], Helga Zoega [1,3], Tracey-Lea Laba [4], Christopher Etherton-Beer [5], Frank M. Sanfilippo [5], Alice Morgan [6], Lisa Kalisch Ellett [2], Claudia Bruno [1], Erin Kelty [5], Maarten IJzerman [7], David B. Preen [5], Claire M. Vajdic [1] and David Henry [8]

[1] Centre for Big Data Research in Health, Faculty of Medicine and Health, UNSW Sydney, Sydney 2052, Australia; j.costa@unsw.edu.au (J.d.O.C.); h.zoega@unsw.edu.au (H.Z.); c.bruno@unsw.edu.au (C.B.); claire.vajdic@unsw.edu.au (C.M.V.)
[2] Quality Use of Medicines and Pharmacy Research Centre, Clinical and Health Sciences, University of South Australia, Adelaide 5000, Australia; nicole.pratt@unisa.edu.au (N.P.); lisa.kalisch@unisa.edu.au (L.K.E.)
[3] Centre of Public Health Sciences, Faculty of Medicine, University of Iceland, 102 Reykjavik, Iceland
[4] Centre for Health Economics Research and Evaluation, Faculty of Health, University of Technology Sydney, Sydney 2006, Australia; Tracey.Laba@chere.uts.edu.au
[5] WA Centre for Health and Ageing, Medical School, University of Western Australia, Perth 6009, Australia; Christopher.Etherton-Beer@uwa.edu.au (C.E.-B.); frank.sanfilippo@uwa.edu.au (F.M.S.); erin.kelty@uwa.edu.au (E.K.); david.preen@uwa.edu.au (D.B.P.)
[6] Research School of Population Health, College of Health and Medicine, Australian National University, Canberra 2601, Australia; alice.morgan@anu.edu.au
[7] Centre for Cancer Research and Centre for Health Policy, Melbourne School of Population and Global Health, University of Melbourne, Melbourne 3000, Australia; maarten.ijzerman@unimelb.edu.au
[8] Institute for Evidence Based Healthcare, Bond University, Gold Coast 4229, Australia; dhenry@bond.edu.au
* Correspondence: sallie.pearson@unsw.edu.au

Abstract: Australia spends more than $20 billion annually on medicines, delivering significant health benefits for the population. However, inappropriate prescribing and medicine use also result in harm to individuals and populations, and waste of precious health resources. Medication data linked with other routine collections enable evidence generation in pharmacoepidemiology; the science of quantifying the use, effectiveness and safety of medicines in real-world clinical practice. This review details the history of medicines policy and data access in Australia, the strengths of existing data sources, and the infrastructure and governance enabling and impeding evidence generation in the field. Currently, substantial gaps persist with respect to cohesive, contemporary linked data sources supporting quality use of medicines, effectiveness and safety research; exemplified by Australia's limited capacity to contribute to the global effort in real-world studies of vaccine and disease-modifying treatments for COVID-19. We propose a roadmap to bolster the discipline, and population health more broadly, underpinned by a distinct capability governing and streamlining access to linked data assets for accredited researchers. Robust real-world evidence generation requires current data roadblocks to be remedied as a matter of urgency to deliver efficient and equitable health care and improve the health and well-being of all Australians.

Keywords: prescribing; quality use of medicines; medication safety; pharmacoepidemiology; medication data; data linkage; health outcomes; real-world data; real-world evidence

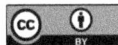

1. Introduction

Prescribing medicines is the most common health intervention globally [1]. Modern medicines have changed the course of major diseases including coronary atherosclerosis, heart failure, stroke, HIV/AIDS and several cancers. However, these major advances have come with costs, both human and financial. Medicines are approved by regulators and payers based on evidence from randomised clinical trials (RCTs) [2,3] but most RCTs are not designed to anticipate, identify, or quantify all possible safety concerns, particularly rare outcomes and long-term effects that only emerge once large numbers of people are exposed over time [4,5]. Moreover, RCTs most commonly focus on single medicines and do not necessarily reflect how medicines are used in patients with complex needs, who require multiple medicines for long periods [4,5]. So, when regulatory and subsidy decisions are made, policy makers, health care professionals, and patients face significant uncertainty about whether the benefits and safety reported in these trials will translate into real-world settings. As such, there is a critical need for rapid and comprehensive evidence about the populations accessing new products, and the benefits and harms associated with their use in routine clinical care.

In addition to generating evidence about the effectiveness and safety of medicines, it is imperative that real-world evidence addresses how medicines are used in routine practice. This is because inappropriate prescribing practices may lead to harm, significant downstream health system burden, and waste of health care resources. In Australia, it is estimated that some 2–3% of all hospital admissions are related to medicine use, rising to 20–30% in people aged 65 years and over [6]. In the period 2016–2017, this equated to ~250,000 hospital admissions, estimated conservatively to cost more than $1.3 billion [6]. Moreover, the high unit cost of some medicines can impact on affordability, resulting in inequities in access and health outcomes.

During the last 20 years, the capacity to generate real-world data on quality use, benefits and safety of prescribed medicines has expanded greatly. The field of pharmacoepidemiology has developed from a primary interest in drug utilisation and ecological exposure-outcome studies to contemporary use of large databases of multiple linked routinely collected, real-world data to estimate the balance between the benefits and harms of medicines [7,8]. These analyses have become increasingly important in decision making. For instance, real-world studies of medicines for COVID-19 have profoundly affected our understanding of the positive and negative impacts of these interventions [9,10]. While insights generated from large databases have the potential to augment our understanding of the impacts of health care interventions, poorly conducted, and even fraudulent studies have important consequences that have led to inappropriate, worthless or harmful treatments being administered to millions of people [11].

Never has there been a more important time to shine the spotlight on Australia's capacity to conduct high-quality, real-world studies of medicine use and effects across a wide range of therapies. In this review, we discuss the use of routine 'medication data' to generate insights and enhance our understanding of the real-world use, benefits and safety of medicines in Australia. In this context, we refer to 'medication data' as an all-encompassing term that includes prescription, dispensing, sales and self-report data about medicine use. Specifically, we will:

- Discuss Australian medicines policies and detail the available medication data that can be leveraged to estimate real-world medicine use;
- Describe how medication data have been used for population-level monitoring, evaluation and research on quality use, effectiveness and safety of medicines, including a COVID-19 case study;
- Highlight the key barriers to delivering a comprehensive research program quantifying real-world use, effectiveness and safety of medicines in Australia; and
- Outline a roadmap to bolster Australia's capacity to accelerate evidence development about effectiveness, safety and quality use of medicines in routine clinical care.

2. Australian Medicines Policies

Australia has a long history of innovation in medicines policies and Australians can access medicines in a variety of ways. They can be prescribed in the community or to patients during hospital stays. Other medicines, including complementary and alternative medicines, can be purchased over the counter (OTC), without a prescription, in community pharmacies or retail stores such as supermarkets.

2.1. National Formulary (The Pharmaceutical Benefits Scheme)

The Pharmaceutical Benefits Scheme (PBS), established in 1948, is a key pillar of Australia's universal health care system, providing all Australian citizens and permanent residents with subsidised access to prescribed medicines [12]. The Repatriation Pharmaceutical Benefits Scheme (RPBS), established in 1919 provides subsidised access to pharmaceuticals to veterans and their dependents. All PBS medicines are available on the RPBS, but eligible veterans' and their dependents have access to additional medicines via the RPBS.

The Pharmaceutical Benefits Advisory Committee (PBAC), formed in the early 1950s, is an independent expert body appointed by the Australian Government recommending new medicines for PBS-listing based on clinical efficacy, safety and cost-effectiveness ('value for money') relative to other available treatments, a process underpinned by RCT evidence. The PBAC pioneered 'value for money' as a pre-requisite for listing in the early 1990s, a process now adopted by governments and third-party payers worldwide [13]. Prior to PBS-listing, a medicine must first be assessed for its quality, efficacy and safety and registered for use in Australia by the Therapeutic Goods Administration (TGA), part of the Australian Government Department of Health. The TGA is responsible for the regulation, registration and ongoing monitoring of medicines safety. Historically, the TGA has relied on periodic review of passive voluntary reports of adverse events from the pharmaceutical industry, prescribers and patients to generate 'signals' for investigation. It is widely acknowledged that this system alone does not meet the needs of a contemporary regulatory system [2,3] and there is a critical need for large-scale and comprehensive post-marketing studies leveraging quality real-world data.

2.2. Quality Use of Medicines (QUM)

The late 1990s and early 2000s also saw the development of pivotal initiatives promoting quality use of medicines (QUM) in Australia. The Australian Government launched the National Medicines Policy [14] and Australia remains one of the few developed countries detailing a comprehensive approach to produce *better health outcomes for all Australians*, focusing on people's access to, and wise use of, medicines. The National Prescribing Service (now *NPS MedicineWise*, Sydney, Australia), a not-for-profit organisation funded by the Commonwealth Department of Health, was launched in 1998. Considered the main implementation arm of the National Medicines Policy, the organisation disseminates evidence-based information and implements educational programs to improve the way in which medicines are prescribed and used in Australia [15]. The *Veterans' Medicines Advice and Therapeutics Education Services* (Veterans' MATES, Adelaide, Australia) program commenced in 2004 to improve the use of medicines and health services in the veterans' community through data-driven health interventions directed to both Department of Veterans' Affairs clients and their health care providers [16]. Most recently, QUM and medicines safety was made the 10th National Health Priority Area by the Council of Australian Governments (COAG) Health Council [17], recognising the urgent need for a coordinated national approach in identifying and promoting best-practice models and measuring progress towards reducing medication related harm.

2.3. A Growing Need for Real-World Data

Given Australia's significant investment in prescribed medicines and QUM initiatives it is imperative that real-world medicines use is monitored to ensure appropriate, effective and safe use. This requires access to comprehensive multiple linked datasets and the capability to perform sophisticated analyses using these data. Cooperation and clear, ongoing governance arrangements between government agencies and academic and not-for-profit institutions are needed to achieve these ends. In the following sections, we detail the diversity of data sources and capabilities needed in Australia to achieve this goal.

3. Quantifying Medicines Use in Australia

Australia is replete with medication data to estimate individual- and population-level medicine use, but the available data remain largely unlinked to information that is needed to gain insights into indications for treatment and health outcomes. Primary data collections (e.g., cross-sectional and longitudinal surveys and disease- or medicine-specific registries) and secondary or routinely collected data (e.g., medicine sales, electronic health records, and dispensing claims) have demonstrated utility in describing medicines use in Australia (Table 1). However, the population coverage and the extent of clinical, dosage, and sociodemographic information varies by data source. This poses challenges for comprehensive quantification of medicine use (including, potential underuse, overuse and misuse) across the entire population and especially in population sub-groups, all of which are critical for QUM assessment. For this reason, we limit our discussion in this paper to potentially linkable data from dispensing and prescription records that provide population-wide metrics.

3.1. Data from Dispensing Records

Records generated when PBS or RPBS prescriptions are dispensed in pharmacies are the mainstay of Australia's routinely collected whole of population medication data. These are electronically generated by systems that have low error rates as they record transactions and attract reimbursements for dispensing pharmacies. PBS records have been shown to accurately reflect prescribed medicine use compared to self-reported use and for medicines prescribed and administered in hospital outpatient settings [18,19]. PBS data have proven an invaluable source of information to quantify population-level medicine use and associated outcomes [7,20]. Notwithstanding the strengths and insights that can be generated from data of this kind, they were not established for research purposes and the gaps in, and limitations of, these data to support QUM research must be acknowledged and addressed. For instance, data on indication and directions for use such as the prescribed daily dose are not available in PBS or RPBS records. In some instances, this can be inferred for medicines used for a single indication, with specific patterns of use, or by linking to other data sources. However, researchers are often required to rely on crude approaches to derive estimates for daily doses, adherence, persistence, and concurrent use when analysing these data.

3.2. Data from Health Records

The growth in access to electronic health records (EHRs) has also contributed significantly to the discipline of pharmacoepidemiology [21]. The value of these collections lies in the richness of the longitudinal data they contain across sociodemographic, behavioural (e.g., smoking status, alcohol consumption) and clinical (e.g., diagnostic, laboratory, prescribing and imaging) domains. These systems have high quality records on all prescriptions written (including indications and directions for use), irrespective of whether they are publicly subsidised or paid in full by patients [22]. However, the quality and comprehensiveness of sociodemographic, diagnostic and other clinical information are variable. Australia does not have a population-wide EHR. The Australian Institute of Health and Welfare (AIHW) was funded in 2018 to develop an enduring National Primary Care Data Asset; however, consultation about the establishment of this asset is ongoing [23]. The Australian Digital Health Agency also rolled out the national My Health Record system in 2018. This is a personally controlled digital health information summary that can be accessed by individuals and health care providers and connects clinical and administrative information on medical encounters, hospitalisations, imaging services, prescriptions, and pathology results. While the system undoubtedly has value, particularly the retrieval of medical data from a central repository during an emergency, a framework for secondary use of those data (e.g., for research) has not been implemented [24,25].

There is no shortage of data available in Australia to quantify and track medicines use. However, there is no comprehensive data source capturing the full spectrum of medicines purchased and consumed by Australians. Moreover, quantifying and capturing changes in medicine use as people transition to different health care settings (for example, from hospital into community or residential aged care) are challenging, due to the siloed nature of the available data collections.

Table 1. Data sources estimating individual and population-level medicine use in Australia.

Data Source	Individual-Level	Medicines Captured	Other Data	Examples
Self-report	Yes	Survey specific: prescribed, OTC, complementary, and alternative	Indication for use; medical history, smoking status, BMI, location of residence	Study specific, e.g., National Health Survey, Australian Longitudinal Study on Women's Health (ALSWH), 45 and Up Cohort Study, Bettering the Evaluation of Healthcare (BEACH)
Registries	Yes	Registry for specific medicines or clinical conditions	Indication for use; medical history, pathology, imaging, smoking status, BMI, location of residence	Disease specific, e.g., Australian National Diabetes Audit Longitudinal Register (ANDA-L), Myeloma and Related Diseases Registry (MRDR), Australian Rheumatology Association Database (ARAD), Australian Register of Clinical Registries
Sales	No, aggregate only	Volume of medicine sold to pharmacies, hospitals, supermarkets	Location of sales	Community pharmacy prescriptions, OTC, complementary and alternative medicine sales data, manufacturer sales, hospital sales
PBS and RPBS dispensing	Yes	R/PBS-listed medicines	Indication for some authority-required medicines, age, sex, beneficiary status, locations of prescriber, pharmacy and beneficiary	PBS and RPBS dispensed medicines from hospital and community pharmacies
Electronic health records	Yes	Medicines administered to hospital in-patients or medicines prescribed in primary care	Indication for use, medical history, pathology, imaging, smoking status, BMI	Hospital: Electronic hospital medication management systems, Hospital discharge summaries Community: General practice clinical software, e.g., Medicine Insight, Melbourne East Monash General Practice Database (MAGNET), GP Population Level Analysis and Reporting (POLAR) Both: My Health Record
Drug surveillance	Yes	Controlled substances	Indication available sometimes	Monitoring of Drugs of Dependence System (MODDS), NSW Controlled Drugs Data Collection (CoDDaC), Real-Time Prescription Monitoring (RTPM)

BMI, body mass index; OTC, over the counter; PBS, Pharmaceutical Benefit Scheme; RPBS, Repatriation Pharmaceutical Benefits Scheme.

3.3. Difficulties Accessing Linked Person-Level Data in Australia

Maximising the value of Australia's health data for comprehensive understanding of QUM and real-world effectiveness and safety of medicines has also had many challenges. At the heart of this issue is timely data access. Complexities arising from cross-jurisdictional data linkage across the Commonwealth, States and Territories and concerns about personal privacy are at the heart of the problem and have impacted significantly on the accessibility and timeliness of these data to generate pharmacoepidemiological research to inform medicines policy development in Australia. The federated health system, where the Commonwealth or States and Territories are responsible for specific aspects of care, means some health data collections are under the custodianship of different agencies across different jurisdictions with different legislation. To undertake comprehensive research on medicine effects, medicines exposure data held by the Commonwealth must be linked with outcomes of interest such as hospitalisation or mortality data that are under State and Territory custodianship. While Australia has invested heavily in its data linkage capability, with data linkage units in all jurisdictions [26] and a cross-jurisdictional capability, we have recently highlighted the complex multi-jurisdictional governance processes that limit comprehensive access to linked health data in Australia [27].

4. Applications of Medication Data in Australia

4.1. Tracking Prescription Medicines Expenditure and Use

The most comprehensive figures on medicine expenditures in Australia, generated by the AIHW, show an annual spend of over $22 billion on prescribed and OTC medicines in the period 2017–2018 for a population of 25 million individuals (this figure includes spending by government, the non-government sector and individuals) [28]. PBS medicines accounted for $11.9 billion of total expenditure; medicines prescribed to public hospital in-patients, private prescriptions and OTC purchases accounted for the remainder. Approximately half of the $3.7 billion spent on medicines purchased OTC was for complementary and alternative medicines. These high-level aggregate figures, however, do not provide insights about individual-level medicine use or QUM. Our recent analysis using individual-level PBS claims in 2018 estimated more than 35% Australians are taking at least one prescribed medicine daily and almost 10% are taking five or more daily [29]. These estimates under-ascertain overall medicine use in our population as they do not include private prescriptions, in-hospital, OTC and complementary and alternative medicines; however, they do generate insights from Australia's largest publicly funded scheme. These analyses and the analytic code underpinning these estimates could be applied to the most contemporary PBS data to generate publicly available up-to-date snapshots of Australian medicine for the information of governments, researchers and the general public.

4.2. Population-Level Monitoring and Evaluation

Many Australian government agencies use medication data routinely to monitor population-level medicine use and outcomes (Table 2). The Drug-Utilisation Sub-Committee (DUSC) of the PBAC was established in 1989 to monitor medicines use post-subsidy (particularly in the first 2 years after PBS listing) and to address specific issues related to QUM. For a period of approximately 20 years DUSC published an annual report, *The Australian Statistics on Medicines (ASM)*, estimating total community use of prescribed medicines (i.e., prescribing outside public hospitals) and detailing prescriptions dispensed according to individual PBS items. Underpinning the publication was a database comprising prescriptions submitted to Medicare Australia for payment of a PBS or RPBS subsidy and estimates of non-subsidised prescriptions; the latter being PBS prescriptions that are under the PBS general beneficiary co-payment and private prescriptions. Estimates of the non-subsidised market were derived from a regular survey of community pharmacies conducted by the Pharmacy Guild of Australia. However, this survey ceased during 2012, coinciding with the collection of unit-record data on under co-payment PBS prescriptions. The last ASM was published in 2016. Since 2003, the Australian Department of Health has generated reports on the number of PBS prescriptions dispensed annually and the total cost to government. However, this is not at the same level of granularity as the ASM, with only the most frequently dispensed PBS medicines and medication classes monitored over consecutive years [30].

Table 2. Government monitoring and evaluation activities.

Activity and Examples (in Italics)	Purpose	Medication Data Used
Medicines use (volume, cost) *Drug-Utilisation Sub-Committee (DUSC) of the PBAC; PBS expenditure and prescriptions reports; AIHW*	Tracks changes in volume of medicines dispensed and total expenditure	PBS and RPBS claims, surveys
QUM interventions and evaluation *NPS MedicineWise; Veterans' MATES*	Improvements in quality of prescribing, improved health outcomes	PBS and RPBS claims, MedicineInsight data
Variations in medicine use *Atlas of Healthcare Variation*	Examine unwarranted variations in use by geographic location	PBS and RPBS claims
Appropriateness of medicine use *Antimicrobial Use and Resistance in Australia (AURA) Surveillance System; Real-Time Prescription Monitoring (RTPM); Prescription Shopping Program*	Reduce inappropriate prescribing, use and associated harms	PBS and RPBS claims, National Antimicrobial Prescribing Survey, National Antimicrobial Utilisation Surveillance Program, MedicineInsight data

PBAC, Pharmaceutical Benefits Scheme Advisory Committee; PBS, Pharmaceutical Benefits Scheme; RPBS, Repatriation Pharmaceutical Benefits Scheme; QUM, Quality Use of Medicines.

The DVA (through their Veterans' MATES program) and NPS MedicineWise use medication data to target feedback to prescribers to improve QUM. Both programs have demonstrated that these interventions have led to improved medicines use and health outcomes [16,31]. The AIHW also uses a wide range of health data, including PBS, to generate authoritative information and statistics on health and welfare topics. It publishes contemporary snapshots of medicine use, like those cited in the previous section of this review.

The Australian Commission on Safety and Quality in Health Care (ACSQHC) uses PBS and RPBS data to generate the Australian Atlas of Healthcare Variation, monitoring and making recommendations to curtail unwarranted variations in medicine use [32–34]. The ACSQHC also hosts the Antimicrobial Use and Resistance in Australia (AURA) Surveillance System, using medication data from various sources to monitor the rate and appropriateness of antimicrobial use in Australia.

The Australian Government National Real-Time Prescription Monitoring (RTPM) system is administered by health departments in each State and Territory. It provides prescribers and pharmacists with up-to-date histories of patients' supply and prescription of controlled substances, including pain medicines such as oxycodone, morphine and fentanyl and other high-risk medicines (determined within each Australian State or Territory), including all benzodiazepines such as diazepam [35]. In addition, the national Prescription Shopping Program provides doctors with data about patients who are at risk of harm because they have multiple medicines prescribed by different doctors.

4.3. Limitations of Current Use of Medication Data in Monitoring and Evaluation

While there is an abundance of activity leveraging medication data across government to monitor the success of Australia's policies, it is striking that they have focused almost solely on estimating and reporting medicine use based on volume and cost. Consequently, assessment or routine reporting about whether this significant investment delivers better health outcomes for our population, as stipulated in our National Medicines Policy, is lacking [14]. Key exceptions are the programs delivered by Veterans' MATES and NPS MedicineWise. In the following sections, we explore the challenges in delivering comprehensive evaluation of the impact of medicine.

5. Medication Data for Research

Internationally, the scientific discipline of pharmacoepidemiology has burgeoned over the last 20 years, driven by a growing interest in the generation of evidence of real-world effects of medicines and assisted by improved access to individual-level linked health data and methods supporting robust causal inferences from those data [5,36–39]. Initially, studies focused on serious adverse effects of specific medicine classes, for instance anti-inflammatory agents and antimicrobials. However, continuing improvements in analytic techniques to reduce selection biases and confounding have enabled studies that estimate treatment benefits equivalent to those seen in large RCTs [40,41].

Characteristics of Australian Pharmacoepidemiological Research Studies

Our systematic reviews [7,20] cataloguing peer-reviewed publications using PBS claims in the period 1987–2018 demonstrate that the vast majority of Australian pharmacoepidemiology research has used aggregate, unliked individual-level PBS, or RPBS data for utilisation studies or to investigate prescriber practice (guideline concordant) or patient behaviour (adherence to treatment) [42–48]. These studies typically investigated medicines acting on the nervous system (opioids, psychotropics) or for treating cardiovascular disease (statins, antihypertensives, and antithrombotics). Many of these studies have been undertaken in DVA clients or people receiving government benefits exclusively (e.g., PBS concessional beneficiaries). However, studies using the entire PBS-eligible population have increased with the availability of under co-payment data in the PBS collections since 2012. Moreover, the number of studies using individual-level PBS data has accelerated in the last decade due to the availability, to the research community, of a standardised, de-identified data collection of person-level dispensing claims for a 10% sample of PBS eligible people ("PBS 10%") [7].

Table 3 details published research using PBS claims to assess medicine-related outcomes. We included the studies identified in our previous systematic reviews and also updated the literature searches, using the same methods, to identify medicine-use outcome studies published in 2019 and 2020. Our synthesis of the 107 studies published from 1987 to 2020 identified two main methodological approaches to assess health outcomes associated with medicine use (see the Supplementary File S1 for the list of included studies). First, ecological studies using aggregated data, whereby trends in medicines use were correlated with trends in outcome rates within the same population. This meant that they assessed population-level outcomes rather than examining individual effects of medicines. The ecological studies investigated clinical outcomes, such as mortality, overdose and poisoning, and were most often generated from publicly available data. Second, studies based on person-level and linked data, which addressed medicines safety outcomes such as infections, development of other health conditions, birth defects, hospitalisations (e.g., for myocardial infarction, pneumonia, falls, and fractures, and death) [49–53]. Studies examining effectiveness measured mostly survival or hospitalisations for specific conditions (e.g., heart failure rehospitalisation following post-discharge beta-blocker initiation) [54].

Over half of the studies leveraging individual-level data were undertaken in the DVA population. As a single payer for all health services provided to their clients, the necessary individual-level medicine exposure and outcomes data are readily available without the need for the complex and time-consuming linkage of data across jurisdictions. While these studies have generated important insights about medicine-related safety they are mostly limited to older Australians and focused primarily on medicines used commonly in older populations such as those acting on the nervous (43%) and cardiovascular (22%) systems. Population-based studies exploring medicine use and outcomes according to Aboriginal and Torres Strait Islander status or for people with a disability, from culturally and linguistically diverse (CaLD) backgrounds and refugees are notably absent. Importantly, Australian data have been used in six [38,55–59] global studies investigating medicine-related health outcomes, using novel statistical techniques that evaluate the sequence of medicines dispensed to identify medicine-adverse events. Another 26 have focused on utilisation patterns to benchmark medicine use in Australia against other countries, such as medicines for attention-deficit hyperactivity disorder (ADHD) [44], antipsychotics [60], and antiepileptics [61].

Table 3. Characteristics of Australian studies assessing medicine use and health outcomes (1987–2020).

Characteristic	Studies Using Aggregate Data ($N = 28$) n (%)	Studies Using Individual-Level Data ($N = 79$) n (%)
Outcome of interest [§]		
Safety (at least one outcome)	26 (92.9)	65 (82.3)
Mortality	12 (42.9)	8 (10.1)
Hospitalisations	5 (17.9)	37 (46.8)
Overdose or poisoning	11 (39.3)	0 (0.0)
Maternal or birth complications	0 (0.0)	8 (10.1)
Other health events	9 (32.1)	21 (26.6)
Effectiveness (at least one outcome)	2 (7.1)	14 (17.7)
Survival	0 (0.0)	9 (11.4)
Hospitalisations	0 (0.0)	4 (5.1)
Health events	2 (7.1)	2 (2.5)
Data sources		
Dispensing claims only	0 (0.0)	12 (15.2)
Dispensing claims and other health data	28 (100.0)	0 (0.0)
Dispensing claims and other linked health data	0 (0.0)	67 (84.8)
Medicines focus according to ATC level [§]		
Alimentary tract and metabolism	1 (3.6)	16 (20.3)
Blood and blood forming organs	1 (3.6)	4 (5.1)
Cardiovascular system	3 (10.7)	17 (21.5)
Genito-urinary system and sex hormones	3 (10.7)	7 (8.9)
Systemic hormonal preparations	0 (0.0)	3 (3.8)
Anti-infectives for systemic use	0 (0.0)	2 (2.5)
Antineoplastic and immunomodulating agents	2 (7.1)	9 (11.4)
Antineoplastic	0 (0.0)	8 (10.1)
Immunomodulating agents	2 (7.1)	1 (1.3)
Musculoskeletal system	3 (10.7)	11 (13.9)
Nervous system	14 (50.0)	34 (43.0)
Respiratory system	0 (0.0)	7 (8.9)
Other ATC groups	0 (0.0)	8 (10.1)
All ATC groups	1 (3.6)	13 (59.1)
Publication Year		
1987–2000	1 (3.6)	0 (0.0)
2001–2005	0 (0.0)	1 (1.3)
2006–2010	7 (25.0)	13 (16.5)
2011–2015	8 (28.6)	30 (38.0)
2016–2020	12 (42.9)	36 (45.6)
Study Population: Age profile		
No age restrictions	24 (85.7)	18 (22.8)
Older adults (≥65 years)	0 (0.0)	46 (58.2)
Adults (≥18 years)	3 (10.7)	4 (5.1)
Women of child-bearing age	0 (0.0)	10 (12.7)
Children *	1 (3.6)	1 (1.3)
Study population: Beneficiary status		
All PBS beneficiaries	24 (85.7)	25 (31.6)
Concessional PBS beneficiaries [†]	4 (14.3)	9 (11.4)
Clients of the Department of Veterans' Affairs	0 (0.0)	45 (57.0)

[§] Study could be classified under more than one category. * Studies also included adolescents or young adults. [†] People receiving government benefits and eligible to pay lower PBS co-payment thresholds. PBS, Pharmaceutical Benefits Scheme.

By international standards the number of individual-level medicine use and outcomes studies conducted in Australia is small [37] and certainly not delivering on its potential given the wealth of data available in this country. Nor does this align with the central tenet of Australia's National Medicines Policy, ensuring we are delivering better health outcomes for our population. We lag far behind other jurisdictions who have joined forces to deliver large-scale global studies of medicine effects to support the evidentiary needs of regulators and payers [62–64]. The case study in Box 1 clearly demonstrates how our current infrastructure and data access operating models are ill-equipped to respond rapidly to emerging questions around the real-world impact of repurposed or newly developed treatments to prevent and manage COVID-19.

Box 1. Australian medication data in the spotlight: Lessons from the COVID-19 pandemic.

The escalating SARS-CoV-2 case numbers worldwide have highlighted the urgent need for timely, robust evidence about the impact of repurposed or newly developed treatments to prevent and manage COVID-19. Evidence from RCTs evaluating the efficacy and safety of vaccines and disease-modifying agents is accumulating [65,66]. However, the speed of emerging viral variants and the related clinical and policy questions about therapies far outpace the capability to conduct new trials and deliver timely answers to these pressing questions. Moreover, each jurisdiction is unique in terms of disease incidence, vaccination availability and uptake, medicine access, prescriber preferences and policy responses. As such, even when trial evidence is published, it is imperative to track the use of these therapies and quantify their effectiveness and harms as they are rolled out across health systems globally. To achieve this, jurisdictions need robust and agile data infrastructure linking individual-level prescription (or dispensing) data to COVID-19 notifications, hospital data, vaccine and death registries plus accurate, meaningful sociodemographic information to inform efficient and equitable public health responses.

Despite the growth in high-quality, real-world evidence addressing emergent clinical questions about vaccines and medicines across the globe [67–69], Australia has been silent on these issues. While some Australian population-based studies are emerging around the changes in prescribed medicine use during the pandemic [70–75], none address questions of significant public interest regarding the effectiveness and safety of therapies for COVID-19. This issue has become even more pressing with the emergence of the SARS-CoV-2 Delta and Omicron variants. In the UK, for example, researchers and analysts at Public Health England produce regularly updated high-quality studies answering these critical questions at a national level [76,77]. In Australia, we have all the data elements necessary to conduct these studies, including a newly established national COVID-19 registry [78], but the data required to address these questions remain unlinked and out of reach of health agencies and researchers.

Below, we highlight some further pressing questions regarding the risk factors, clinical progress, prevention, amelioration and treatment of infections by the SARS-CoV-2 variants.

(1) What are the current major determinants of risk of developing severe disease after infection with the Delta variant? How is this changing over time and how do the risk factors compare with the earlier viral strains?
(2) What proportion of patients suffering from COVID-19, and being managed in the community, are receiving adequate evidence-based treatments?
(3) How many individuals receiving unproven, in effective or harmful COVID-19 treatments? This includes, but is not limited to, ivermectin, azithromycin, vitamin D, zinc and quinine derivatives.
(4) What are the socioeconomic factors that determine access to vaccines and how can these population sub-groups most rapidly and effectively be targeted?
(5) How well are the current vaccines (Pfizer, AstraZeneca, and Moderna) working against the Delta virus strain in Australia (in preventing infection, transmission, hospitalisation, ICU admission and death)?
(6) What is the comparative safety of the AstraZeneca and mRNA vaccines (Pfizer and Moderna) in terms of acute sensitivity reactions, thrombocytopenia/venous thrombosis, heart attacks, strokes and myocarditis? In Australia, how do these vaccine-associated risks compare with the risks of acquiring COVID-19?
(7) How should the limited supply of new and expensive monoclonal antibody treatments, now available for treatment of mild to moderate COVID-19 outside hospital, be targeted to those most likely to benefit? Should they be combined with other therapies, e.g., inhaled or oral corticosteroids?
(8) Will the early use of monoclonal antibodies in Australia reduce pressure on the hospital systems?

As a matter of urgency, we propose the creation of a resilient data infrastructure [79] needed to address the questions outlined above. This will enable researchers and governments to respond rapidly to emerging information needs around the evolving pandemic and other major public health challenges.

The pandemic has heightened the aspirations of the international pharmacoepidemiology community to provide much needed evidence in this global public health crisis. However, the publication of poor-quality studies, some of which are based on fraudulent or flawed data, has also exacerbated criticisms that studies of this kind are not reliable or trustworthy [10]. Robust data infrastructure is a key building block to deliver evidence complementing RCTs, however, this must be accompanied by international best-practice principles of transparent and reproducible reporting.

6. Key Barriers to Delivering a Comprehensive Program on Real-World Use, Effectiveness and Safety of Medicines in Australia

Our analysis of the peer-reviewed literature examining the outcomes associated with PBS medicine use clearly demonstrates the mismatch between Australia's annual multi-billion-dollar investment in prescribed medicines and capability to deliver a comprehensive program evaluating the health benefits and harms derived from this investment. There have been a series of high-profile reviews, including the Productivity Commission Report on Data Availability and Use [80] and the Senate Select Committee on Health Sixth Interim Report, Big Health Data: Australia's Big Potential [81] documenting the contemporary challenges facing the research, government and business sectors in realising the potential of Australian data and recommending responses to turn this situation around (Box 2).

Box 2. Historical challenges to data availability and use in Australia and key recommendations (dot points) from the Productivity Commission and Senate Select Committee on Health.

Privacy and data access concerns and lack of trust in existing data access processes and protections
• Develop risk-based data access framework based on risks associated with different types of data, uses of data and use environments
• Ensure linkage policies and regulations are developed to world's best-practice standard
Legal, institutional and technical barriers
• Simplify existing legislative framework for data access, standardise data sharing agreements, including those pertinent to States and Territories
• Accredit State and Territory, in addition to Commonwealth, data linkage units to link Commonwealth data with State data collections, subject to comprehensive privacy and security protocols
• Use an open data policy for low-risk de-identified data collections
Lengthy, complex and inefficient approval processes and a culture of risk aversion
• Establish new statutory office holder, with responsibility for enabling effective use of data, oversight, guidance and updating operations
• Designate national interest datasets to enable wider use across and between sectors (public, private, not-for-profit and academia) and jurisdictions
• Increase transparency around government data holdings including clear statements regarding dataset approval processes
• By default, deidentified datasets should be released on an enduring basis
Duplicative efforts of ethics committees
• Reform ethics processes including registration requirements and mutual recognition of approvals from accredited jurisdictions
Costs
• Develop enduring linked data assets for use by multiple end-users including government, researchers and other third parties

In the five years since the publication of these recommendations, the Office of the National Data Commissioner has been established and enabled legislation in the form of the Data Availability and Transparency (DAT) Bill 2020 currently before parliament. The purpose of this Bill is to:

- Implement a scheme authorising and regulating access to Australian Government data (this does not include data collected by State and Territory Governments or My Health Record);
- Authorise public-sector data custodians to share data with accredited users according to specific authorisations, purposes, principles and agreements;
- Establish and specify the functions and powers of the National Data Commissioner as the regulator of the scheme and the National Data Advisory Council as an advisory body to the commissioner; and
- Establish the regulation and enforcement framework for the scheme.

The Bill will be a key enabler to data access and use. However, the timeline as well as ways in which the legislation will be interpreted and implemented remain uncertain. Key to this endeavour is sharing of data across jurisdictional boundaries. While almost every Australian jurisdiction has data sharing pathways in place, they vary in their levels of maturity. In a forward step in July 2021, an intergovernmental agreement on data sharing between Commonwealth, State and Territory governments was signed committing all governments to share data between jurisdictions as a default position, if it can be done securely, safely, lawfully and ethically [82]. While this agreement should provide impetus to improve access across jurisdictional boundaries, it makes no reference to data sharing and use for research. This should be remedied.

6.1. Tentative Steps towards Greater Data Access in Australia

New guidance is emerging based on the Five Safes Framework, an internationally recognised approach assessing strategic, privacy, security, ethical and operational risks associated with data sharing or release [83]. The DAT Bill 2020 refers to Data Sharing Principles modelled on the Five Safes Framework. However, the Framework is principles based, and subject to interpretation at the coal face. This results in significant heterogeneity and inconsistency between policy agencies. For data linkage projects, this creates lengthy delays and considerable burdens on data custodians and end-users applying for access. It is well documented that data governance demands and inadequate resourcing within government to directly support data access remain as major challenges to research in this area [81]. Data safe havens that securely house potentially sensitive data are a fundamental pillar of the Framework. The ABS DataLab, the Department of Health's Enterprise Data Warehouse (EDW), the AIHW Secure Remote Access Environment (SRAE), E-Research Institutional Cloud Architecture (ERICA), and the Sax Institute's Secure Unified Research Environment (SURE) are examples of these facilities. However, resilient remote-access facilities with fit-for-purpose infrastructure and administrative policies and procedures are yet to be delivered at scale.

6.2. Inefficiencies in Ethics Approvals for Research Using Linked Data

The Australian National Health and Medical Research Council (NHMRC) Statement on the Ethical Conduct in Human Research [84] has recently been refreshed and provides explicit, implementable guidance on database and data linkage research. However, there is not yet a national approach to single HREC review for data linkage research. While Australian State and Territory health departments have signed a Memorandum of Understanding for mutual acceptance of ethical and scientific review of multi-centre human research projects undertaken in public health organisations, projects involving access to state-wide data collections from every jurisdiction are not included, meaning researchers must navigate duplicative and often inconsistent requirements to gain approval for data linkage studies. Therefore, health data linkage research continues to lag behind other forms of health research including clinical trials of new therapies, resulting in inefficiencies, duplicated effort, inconsistencies and research waste. The challenges with HREC inefficiencies notwithstanding, the major impediment to timely data access, linkage and use are deficient data governance processes.

6.3. Tentative Steps to Create National Linked Data Assets

There have been encouraging moves to develop multi-source enduring linked data assets (MELDAs) of national significance. One key example, that could deliver important insights relating to real-world quality use of medicines, safety and effectiveness research, is the National Integrated Health Services Information (NIHSI) asset [85], developed by and under the custodianship of the AIHW. However, several years on from its establishment, formal policies around third-party access, including to academic researchers, are yet to be established. While this asset has been leveraged within government and NIHISI's precursor (the National Data Linkage Demonstration Project) was accessed by researchers, they were acting as contractors to government. Despite its great promise, the outputs from this resource have been limited to a few publicly available publications and government reports [86–88]. The end result is a situation where (i) considerable government investment has been made to create data resource that is not maximally used, and (ii) a highly trained and skilled workforce is unable to access these valuable and comprehensive enduring linked data for the public good.

7. Recommendations to Bolster Australia's Capacity to Accelerate Evidence Development about Quality Use, Effectiveness and Safety of Medicines in Routine Clinical Care

Box 3 outlines our key recommendations to accelerate pharmacoepidemiological research in Australia and leverage the large and growing volumes of routinely collected data to generate evidence for regulators, payers, clinicians, and patients about how medicines are used and how they perform outside the narrow confines of RCTs.

Box 3. Recommendations to bolster pharmacoepidemiological research in Australia.

Scale up and streamline data access and use
• Generate publicly available, contemporary snapshots of Australian medicines use
• Increase availability and streamline access to population-wide PBS unit-record data
• Establish dedicated enduring cross-jurisdictional linked data with access for non-government researchers
Enhance medication data collections
• Include private prescriptions in national dispensing data collections
• Link population-wide dispensing and other administrative data to electronic health records

Our review has highlighted the need to deliver publicly available, contemporary Australian statistics on medicines in a user-friendly, interactive form. This will create new levels of transparency for all QUM stakeholders and significantly reduce the burden of bespoke data requests to the custodians of medication data. Starting with PBS and RPBS data, we need to move beyond simple volume and cost metrics and report person-centric information such as number of people dispensed a specific medicine over a defined period (this could be to the level of PBS item codes). Other jurisdictions, such as Denmark, have paved the way for medicine statistics [89], publicly reporting information on prescribed and OTC medicines dispensed/sold, which can be stratified by year, sex, age groups, geographical area (region) and sector (primary or secondary health care sector).

We also demonstrated, in our catalogue of peer-reviewed research using PBS claims, that the availability of a standardised collection of longitudinal person-level PBS data has contributed to the rapid increase in the number of studies investigating QUM, particularly for those used widely in the community. Available via a contract with Services Australia, the collection dates back to 2005 and is now updated monthly and includes the dispensing history for a 10% sample of PBS-eligible Australians. We strongly advocate for this collection to be scaled up to support robust analyses for all PBS medicines; many of the high-cost medicines available on the PBS are for distinct patient sub-groups (e.g., targeted cancer therapies). The current collection is not fit-for-purpose to examine QUM in these high-cost but relatively small volume therapeutic areas.

To bolster high-quality pharmacoepidemiology research, Australian researchers require access to enduring collections of cross-jurisdictional linked data. We support the establishment of an enduring, regularly updated collection linking, at a minimum, PBS, Medicare Benefits Scheme, hospitalisation, emergency department, cancer, and death records; this collection is essentially the NIHSI with the addition of cancer registry data. While this will not negate the need for purpose-built collections, it will serve a substantive proportion of the pharmacoepidemiological research needs. Over time, such a linkage could be augmented with other medication data and routine data collections. For example, access to individual-level dispensing records for private as well as publicly subsidised prescriptions will support more comprehensive QUM reporting, particularly co-prescribing and multi-medicine use. Moreover, linkage to prescribing data held in primary care electronic health records will provide information about all medicines prescribed (not just those that are publicly subsidised), the indication for prescribing, prescribed daily dose and intended duration of therapy. Coupling dispensing and prescribing data expands opportunities to explore critical issues such as primary non-adherence—when prescriptions are written but never filled [90]. Data enhancements enabling researchers to more accurately identify important population sub-groups will enable sophisticated analyses of social and economic determinants of health [91]. All of these enhancements will enable timely and cost-effective responses to new threats to public health and safety; the situation highlighted in our COVID-19 case study needs to be remedied as a matter of urgency.

8. Liberating Australia's Linked Health Data Assets

In this review, we concentrated primarily on enhancements pertaining directly to QUM and pharmacoepidemiological research. We recognise that pharmacoepidemiology sits within a broader discipline of population health research. Box 4 details a series of recommendations that will bolster Australian population health research more broadly and also benefit the discipline of pharmacoepidemiology. In this context, Australia could learn from mature population health research operating models overseas.

Box 4. Recommendations to bolster population health research (including pharmacoepidemiology) in Australia.

Establish a distinct capability governing and streamlining access to linked data assets for accredited researchers
• Convene single independent scientific and ethical review of projects leveraging key data collections
• Centralise governance review on behalf of original data custodians
Promote transparency and reproducibility
• Ensure research protocols, analytical code, and data outputs are disseminated freely and openly
Standardise data and analytic tools
• Use common data models, vocabularies and coding
Build and maintain public trust
• Demonstrate the value of data, including enduring linked assets, to improve health system efficiency and equity and the health and well-being of ALL Australians

8.1. International Models for Centralisation and Separation of Data Access for Policy and Research

Mature population health research capabilities in jurisdictions such as the United Kingdom, the European Union and Canada, have evolved differently, but they have some common elements Australia would be wise to adopt to scale up current capabilities [92,93]. They all promote the exchange and access to different types of health data for research, have transparent data governance, data sharing agreements for the specific purpose of research and foster continuous improvements around data quality and interoperability. Critically, they have all created distinct entities managing linked data access for approved researchers, essentially separating data provision for routine reporting functions and informing health policy from research. We believe that centralisation of linked health data in Australian government agencies is appropriate, important and should continue for statistical monitoring, and reporting activities. While agencies such as the Australian Bureau of Statistics (ABS) and AIHW have advanced capabilities and capacity to deliver on many of these functions, they are currently not sufficiently equipped or funded to provide the resources and expertise to meet the contemporary research and evaluation needs of a contemporary federated health system. Moreover, these agencies do not have the capacity and resources to manage the substantial number of data requests for the research community. This is likely to become more acute once the enabling legislation is passed and other long-standing roadblocks detailed in Box 2 have been resolved.

8.2. A Roadmap for Australia

A more contemporary operating model for Australian population health research would establish a distinct capability with the primary purpose of data access and use for accredited researchers. Aligning with other approaches internationally, this could be delivered by an independent entity or entities. The capability would function strictly according to the Five Safes principles, satisfy legislative requirements at both Commonwealth, State and Territory levels and at arm's length to vested interests, political, commercial or other. The capability would require up-front government investment but be implemented with a user-pays pricing model. This proposed operating model aligns with the current Australian data reforms and will enhance research and innovation in population health and reduce the significant amounts of research dollars currently invested in the highly convoluted and slow data linkage landscape.

Under this operating model, existing Accredited Data Authorities would continue their work integrating data across jurisdictional boundaries, but they would provide the new capabilities with the core data infrastructure and receive regular data feeds to update the data for the population they are serving. The data provider would also have a key accountability for transparent and efficient response times, a fundamental requirement for publicly funded research. Moreover, a common data model would be integral to the approach, transforming data into common formats using standardised terminologies and vocabularies. Common data models are rapidly accelerating large-scale population health research across the globe as they facilitate systematic data interrogation using libraries of standard analytic routines [64,94]. Critically, the independent capability would assume responsibility as the data custodian of their holdings, absolving the original data custodians of responsibilities for the downstream use of the data. They would undertake single, independent scientific and ethical review of projects leveraging their data holdings; this would obviate the need for ethical and scientific review of projects by multiple jurisdictional entities.

Data sharing agreements with researchers would specify the range of proposed uses for the data, that data should never be reidentified and that data can never be downloaded from its secure host site or in a format that allows identification of individuals. All analyses and products of the analyses would be risk-assessed before release to researchers for use in publications and other scientific outputs. As a condition of data release, the capability would require research projects to align with the international best-practice principles of transparent reporting to ensure all sectors, including the Australian public, have readily accessible information about the approved uses and products of data access. This could take the form of an open, publicly available register using standardised protocol templates [95,96], similar to the long-standing practice of RCT registration. This level of transparency also advances the goal of reproducibility and facilitates peer-review.

Finally, the capabilities will also have a responsibility for, and play a pivotal role in, maintaining public trust, communicating and educating stakeholders about the benefits (and potential risks) of using data for the public good. Fundamental to this effort is embedding and implementing equity principles to identify, monitor and reduce socioeconomic, cultural, gender and age inequities in medicine and health service use and outcomes [91].

9. Conclusions

Australia spends in excess of $20 billion annually on medicines. There is no doubt that this has resulted in significant health gains for individuals and populations, but it has also been accompanied by substantial harm and health care costs. Consequently, QUM and medicine safety were announced as Australia's 10th National Health Priority in 2019. Throughout this review, we highlighted the significant mismatch between Australia's annual multi-billion-dollar investment in medicines and our capability to deliver a comprehensive research program evaluating the health benefits and harms derived from this investment. We repeatedly highlighted the deficiencies in data access in Australia and how it lags behind most countries with mature publicly funded health care systems. We pointed to the need to establish centralised or distributed data assets operating under the Five Safes principles which would also support contemporary, collaborative, ethical and reproducible research and government activity in population health. In the context of the COVID-19 pandemic, Australia has been notably absent in the global effort to better understand the real-world impact of repurposed or newly developed treatments to prevent and manage

COVID-19. The establishment of widely accessible national health data assets is now a matter of urgency. We urge decision makers to respond to this challenge.

Supplementary Materials: The following are available online at https://www.mdpi.com/1660-4601/18/24/13345/s1, File S1: Studies included in this review assessing medicine exposure and outcomes using Pharmaceutical Benefits Scheme or Repatriation Pharmaceutical Benefits Scheme data.

Author Contributions: S.-A.P., N.P., D.H., C.M.V. and D.B.P. conceptualised this paper. J.d.O.C. and C.B. undertook the literature search and data extraction for the review of Australian studies leveraging PBS claims. N.P. and S.-A.P. worked with J.d.O.C. and C.B. to catalogue and interpret the literature. S.-A.P., N.P., J.d.O.C., H.Z., T.-L.L., C.E.-B., F.M.S., A.M., L.K.E., C.B., E.K., M.I., D.B.P., C.M.V. and D.H. contributed to the manuscript draft, reviewed and edited the manuscript and approved the final submitted version. All authors have read and agreed to the published version of the manuscript.

Funding: This review is supported by the National Health and Medical Research Council (NHMRC) Centre of Research Excellence in Medicines Intelligence (GNT1196900); H.Z. is supported by a UNSW Scientia Fellowship; E.K. is supported by an NHMRC Emerging Leader Fellowship (APP1172978); C.B. is supported by an Australian Government Research Training Program Scholarship.

Institutional Review Board Statement: Not applicable.

Informed Consent Statement: Not applicable.

Data Availability Statement: Data sharing is not applicable to this article.

Acknowledgments: We would like to thank Barry Sandison for his insightful comments on this manuscript. This paper was written on behalf of the Centre of Research Excellence in Medicines Intelligence investigators; Chief investigators: Sallie-Anne Pearson, Nicole Pratt, Nicholas Buckley, David B. Preen, Louisa Degenhardt, Kees Van Gool, Claire M. Vajdic, Louisa Jorm, Andrew Wilson, David Henry; and Associate Investigators: Anne McKenzie, Christopher Etherton-Beer, Debra Rowett, Frank M. Sanfilippo, Helga Zoega, Julian Elliott, Sarah Lord, Timothy Dobbins, Tracey-Lea Laba, and Ximena Camacho.

Conflicts of Interest: C.E.B. is a member of the Pharmaceutical Benefits Advisory Committee (PBAC); S.P., N.P., T.L. and C.E.B. are members of the Drug-Utilization Sub-Committee of the PBAC; T.L. is a member of the Economics Sub-Committee of the PBAC; M.I. is a member of the Economics Sub-Committee of the MSAC; S.P. is a member of the National Data Advisory Council; C.M.V. is Deputy Chair of the NSW Population Health Service Research Ethics Committee; D.P. is a member of the Sax Institute Board. The views of authors expressed in this review article are their own and do not represent those of the aforementioned bodies. In 2020, the Centre for Big Data Research in Health received funding from AbbVie Australia to conduct post-market surveillance research. AbbVie did not have any knowledge of, or involvement in, this manuscript.

References

1. Aitken, M.; Kleinrock, M. *Global Medicines Use in 2020: Outlook and Implications*; IMS Institute for Healthcare Informatics: Parsippany, NJ, USA, 2015.
2. Kelman, C.W.; Pearson, S.A.; Day, R.O.; Holman, C.D.; Kliewer, E.V.; Henry, D.A. Evaluating medicines: Let's use all the evidence. *Med. J. Aust.* **2007**, *186*, 249–252. [CrossRef]
3. Banks, E.; Pearson, S.A. A life-cycle approach to monitoring benefits and harms of medicines. *Med. J. Aust.* **2012**, *197*, 313–314. [CrossRef] [PubMed]
4. Frieden, T.R. Evidence for Health Decision Making—Beyond Randomized, Controlled Trials. *N. Engl. J. Med.* **2017**, *377*, 465–475. [CrossRef] [PubMed]
5. Avorn, J. In defense of pharmacoepidemiology—Embracing the yin and yang of drug research. *N. Engl. J. Med.* **2007**, *357*, 2219–2221. [CrossRef]
6. Pharmaceutical Society of Australia. *Medicine Safety: Take Care*; PSA: Canberra, Australia, 2019.
7. de Oliveira Costa, J.; Bruno, C.; Schaffer, A.L.; Raichand, S.; Karanges, E.A.; Pearson, S.A. The changing face of Australian data reforms: Impact on pharmacoepidemiology research. *Int. J. Popul. Data Sci.* **2021**, *6*, 1418. [CrossRef]
8. Young, A.; Flack, F. Recent trends in the use of linked data in Australia. *Aust. Health Rev.* **2018**, *42*, 584–590. [CrossRef]
9. Morales, D.R.; Conover, M.M.; You, S.C.; Pratt, N.; Kostka, K.; Duarte-Salles, T.; Fernández-Bertolín, S.; Aragón, M.; DuVall, S.L.; Lynch, K.; et al. Renin-angiotensin system blockers and susceptibility to COVID-19: An international, open science, cohort analysis. *Lancet Digit. Health* **2021**, *3*, e98–e114. [CrossRef]

10. Franklin, J.M.; Lin, K.J.; Gatto, N.M.; Rassen, J.A.; Glynn, R.J.; Schneeweiss, S. Real-World Evidence for Assessing Pharmaceutical Treatments in the Context of COVID-19. *Clin. Pharmacol. Ther.* **2021**, *109*, 816–828. [CrossRef]
11. Benchimol, E.I.; Moher, D.; Ehrenstein, V.; Langan, S.M. Retraction of COVID-19 Pharmacoepidemiology Research Could Have Been Avoided by Effective Use of Reporting Guidelines. *Clin. Epidemiol.* **2020**, *12*, 1403–1420. [CrossRef]
12. Biggs, A. The Pharmaceutical Benefits Scheme—An Overview. Available online: https://www.aph.gov.au/About_Parliament/Parliamentary_Departments/Parliamentary_Library/Publications_Archive/archive/pbs (accessed on 24 August 2021).
13. Birkett, D.J.; Mitchell, A.S.; McManus, P. A cost-effectiveness approach to drug subsidy and pricing in Australia. *Health Aff.* **2001**, *20*, 104–114. [CrossRef]
14. Australian Department of Health and Ageing. *National Medicines Policy 2000*; Commonwealth of Australia: Canberra, Australia, 1999.
15. Weekes, L.M.; Mackson, J.M.; Fitzgerald, M.; Phillips, S.R. National Prescribing Service: Creating an implementation arm for national medicines policy. *Br. J. Clin. Pharmacol.* **2005**, *59*, 112–116. [CrossRef]
16. Australian Government Department of Veterans' Affairs. What is Veterans' MATES? Available online: https://www.veteransmates.net.au/what-is-veterans-mates (accessed on 24 August 2021).
17. Australian Journal of Pharmacy. Don't Stop Here, Ministers: PSA. Available online: https://ajp.com.au/news/dont-stop-there-ministers-psa/ (accessed on 10 September 2021).
18. Gnjidic, D.; Du, W.; Pearson, S.A.; Hilmer, S.N.; Banks, E. Ascertainment of self-reported prescription medication use compared with pharmaceutical claims data. *Public Health Res. Pract.* **2017**, *27*. [CrossRef] [PubMed]
19. Harris, C.; Daniels, B.; Ward, R.L.; Pearson, S.A. Retrospective comparison of Australia's Pharmaceutical Benefits Scheme claims data with prescription data in HER2-positive early breast cancer patients, 2008–2012. *Public Health Res. Pract.* **2017**, *27*, e275174. [CrossRef]
20. Pearson, S.A.; Pesa, N.; Langton, J.M.; Drew, A.; Faedo, M.; Robertson, J. Studies using Australia's Pharmaceutical Benefits Scheme data for pharmacoepidemiological research: A systematic review of the published literature (1987–2013). *Pharmacoepidemiol. Drug. Saf.* **2015**, *24*, 447–455. [CrossRef] [PubMed]
21. Hennessy, S. Use of health care databases in pharmacoepidemiology. *Basic Clin. Pharmacol. Toxicol.* **2006**, *98*, 311–313. [CrossRef]
22. Gordon, J.; Miller, G.; Britt, H. *Reality Check-Reliable National Data from General Practice Electronic Health Records*; Deeble Institute: Sydney, Australia, 2016.
23. Australian Institute of Health and Welfare. *Developing a National Primary Health Care Data Asset: Consultation report. Cat. No. PHC 1*; AIHW: Canberra, Australia, 2019.
24. Australian Digital Health Agency. Fact Sheet: How Secondary Use of My Health Record Data Can Improve Health Outcomes for Australians. Available online: https://www.myhealthrecord.gov.au/sites/default/files/hd315_factsheet_secondary_use_of_data.pdf?v=1535679293. (accessed on 25 August 2021).
25. Canaway, R.; Boyle, D.I.; Manski-Nankervis, J.E.; Bell, J.; Hocking, J.S.; Clarke, K.; Clark, M.; Gunn, J.M.; Emery, J.D. Gathering data for decisions: Best practice use of primary care electronic records for research. *Med. J. Aust.* **2019**, *210* (Suppl. 6), S12–S16. [CrossRef] [PubMed]
26. Flack, F.; Smith, M. The Population Health Research Network—Population Data Centre Profile. *Int. J. Popul. Data Sci.* **2019**, *4*, 1130. [CrossRef]
27. Henry, D.; Stehlik, P.; Camacho, X.; Pearson, S.-A. Access to routinely collected data for population health research: Experiences in Canada and Australia. *Aust. N. Z. J. Public Health* **2018**, *42*, 430–433. [CrossRef] [PubMed]
28. Australian Institute of Health and Welfare. Medicines in the Health System. Available online: https://www.aihw.gov.au/reports/australias-health/medicines-in-the-health-system (accessed on 24 August 2021).
29. Wylie, C.; Daniels, B.; Brett, J.; Pearson, S.A.; Buckley, N.A. A national study on prescribed medicine in Australia on a typical day. *Pharmacoepidemiol. Drug. Saf.* **2020**, *29*, 1046–1053. [CrossRef]
30. PBS Information Management Section; Pricing and PBS Policy Branch; Technology Assessment and Access Division. *PBS Expenditure and Prescriptions Report 1 July 2019 to 30 June 2020*; Department of Health: Canberra, Australia, 2020.
31. NPS MedicineWise. *Creating Impact Together. Annual Report 2020*; NPS MedicineWise: Sydney, Australia, 2020.
32. Australian Commission on Safety and Quality in Health Care; Australian Institute of Health and Welfare. *The Fourth Australian Atlas of Healthcare Variation*; ACSQHC: Sydney, Australia, 2021.
33. Australian Commission on Safety and Quality in Health Care; Australian institute of Health and Welfare. *The Third Australian Atlas of Healthcare Variation*; ACSQHC: Sydney, Australia, 2018.
34. Australian Commission on Safety and Quality in Health Care; National Health Performance Authority. *Australian Atlas of Healthcare Variation*; ACSQHC: Sydney, Australia, 2015.
35. Australian Government Department of Health. National Real Time Prescription Monitoring (RTPM). Available online: https://www.health.gov.au/initiatives-and-programs/national-real-time-prescription-monitoring-rtpm (accessed on 11 August 2021).
36. Schneeweiss, S.; Avorn, J. A review of uses of health care utilization databases for epidemiologic research on therapeutics. *J. Clin. Epidemiol.* **2005**, *58*, 323–337. [CrossRef]
37. Wettermark, B.; Zoëga, H.; Furu, K.; Korhonen, M.; Hallas, J.; Nørgaard, M.; Almarsdottir, A.; Andersen, M.; Andersson Sundell, K.; Bergman, U.; et al. The Nordic prescription databases as a resource for pharmacoepidemiological research—A literature review. *Pharmacoepidemiol. Drug. Saf.* **2013**, *22*, 691–699. [CrossRef] [PubMed]

38. Pratt, N.; Andersen, M.; Bergman, U.; Choi, N.K.; Gerhard, T.; Huang, C.; Kimura, M.; Kimura, T.; Kubota, K.; Lai, E.C.; et al. Multi-country rapid adverse drug event assessment: The Asian Pharmacoepidemiology Network (AsPEN) antipsychotic and acute hyperglycaemia study. *Pharmacoepidemiol. Drug. Saf.* **2013**, *22*, 915–924. [CrossRef] [PubMed]
39. Observational Health Data Sciences and Informatics. OHDSI Studies. Available online: https://data.ohdsi.org/OhdsiStudies/ (accessed on 30 August 2021).
40. Hernán, M.A.; Robins, J.M. Using Big Data to Emulate a Target Trial When a Randomized Trial Is Not Available. *Am. J. Epidemiol.* **2016**, *183*, 758–764. [CrossRef]
41. Labrecque, J.A.; Swanson, S.A. Target trial emulation: Teaching epidemiology and beyond. *Eur. J. Epidemiol.* **2017**, *32*, 473–475. [CrossRef] [PubMed]
42. Karanges, E.A.; Buckley, N.A.; Brett, J.; Blanch, B.; Litchfield, M.; Degenhardt, L.; Pearson, S.A. Trends in opioid utilisation in Australia, 2006–2015: Insights from multiple metrics. *Pharmacoepidemiol. Drug. Saf.* **2018**, *27*, 504–512. [CrossRef] [PubMed]
43. Lee, J.; Pilgrim, J.; Gerostamoulos, D.; Robinson, J.; Wong, A. Increasing rates of quetiapine overdose, misuse, and mortality in Victoria, Australia. *Drug Alcohol Depend.* **2018**, *187*, 95–99. [CrossRef]
44. Raman, S.R.; Man, K.K.C.; Bahmanyar, S.; Berard, A.; Bilder, S.; Boukhris, T.; Bushnell, G.; Crystal, S.; Furu, K.; KaoYang, Y.H.; et al. Trends in attention-deficit hyperactivity disorder medication use: A retrospective observational study using population-based databases. *Lancet Psychiat.* **2018**, *5*, 824–835. [CrossRef]
45. Brett, J.; Daniels, B.; Karanges, E.A.; Buckley, N.A.; Schneider, C.; Nassir, A.; McLachlan, A.J.; Pearson, S.A. Psychotropic polypharmacy in Australia, 2006 to 2015: A descriptive cohort study. *Br. J. Clin. Pharmacol.* **2017**, *83*, 2581–2588. [CrossRef]
46. Daniels, B.; Girosi, F.; Tervonen, H.; Kiely, B.E.; Lord, S.J.; Houssami, N.; Pearson, S.A. Adherence to prescribing restrictions for HER2-positive metastatic breast cancer in Australia: A national population-based observational study (2001–2016). *PLoS ONE* **2018**, *13*, e0198152. [CrossRef]
47. de Oliveira Costa, J.; Schaffer, A.L.; Medland, N.A.; Litchfield, M.; Narayan, S.W.; Guy, R.; McManus, H.; Pearson, S.A. Adherence to Antiretroviral Regimens in Australia: A Nationwide Cohort Study. *AIDS Patient Care STDS* **2020**, *34*, 81–91. [CrossRef]
48. Jones, G.; Hall, S.; Bird, P.; Littlejohn, G.; Tymms, K.; Youssef, P.; Chung, E.; Barrett, R.; Button, P. A retrospective review of the persistence on bDMARDs prescribed for the treatment of rheumatoid arthritis in the Australian population. *Int. J. Rheum. Dis.* **2018**, *21*, 1581–1590. [CrossRef] [PubMed]
49. Colvin, L.; Slack-Smith, L.; Stanley, F.J.; Bower, C. Linking a pharmaceutical claims database with a birth defects registry to investigate birth defect rates of suspected teratogens. *Pharmacoepidemiol. Drug Saf.* **2010**, *19*, 1137–1150. [CrossRef]
50. Lopez, D.; Preen, D.B.; Etherton-Beer, C.; Sanfilippo, F.M. Frailty, and not medicines with anticholinergic or sedative effects, predicts adverse outcomes in octogenarians admitted for myocardial infarction: Population-level study. *Australas. J. Ageing* **2021**, *40*, e155–e162. [CrossRef] [PubMed]
51. Pratt, N.; Roughead, E.E.; Ramsay, E.; Salter, A.; Ryan, P. Risk of hospitalization for hip fracture and pneumonia associated with antipsychotic prescribing in the elderly: A self-controlled case-series analysis in an Australian health care claims database. *Drug Saf.* **2011**, *34*, 567–575. [CrossRef] [PubMed]
52. Castle, D.J.; Chung, E. Cardiometabolic comorbidities and life expectancy in people on medication for schizophrenia in Australia. *Curr. Med. Res. Opin.* **2018**, *34*, 613–618. [CrossRef]
53. Pratt, N.L.; Ramsay, E.; Kalisch Ellett, L.M.; Duszynski, K.; Shakib, S.; Kerr, M.; Caughey, G.; Roughead, E.E. Comparative effectiveness and safety of low-strength and high-strength direct oral anticoagulants compared with warfarin: A sequential cohort study. *BMJ Open* **2019**, *9*, e026486. [CrossRef]
54. Qin, X.; Hung, J.; Knuiman, M.; Teng, T.K.; Briffa, T.; Sanfilippo, F.M. Evidence-based pharmacotherapies used in the postdischarge phase are associated with improved one-year survival in senior patients hospitalized with heart failure. *Cardiovasc. Ther.* **2018**, *36*, e12464. [CrossRef]
55. Lai, E.C.; Shin, J.Y.; Kubota, K.; Man, K.K.C.; Park, B.J.; Pratt, N.; Roughead, E.E.; Wong, I.C.K.; Kao Yang, Y.H.; Setoguchi, S. Comparative safety of NSAIDs for gastrointestinal events in Asia-Pacific populations: A multi-database, international cohort study. *Pharmacoepidemiol. Drug. Saf.* **2018**, *27*, 1223–1230. [CrossRef] [PubMed]
56. Pratt, N.; Chan, E.W.; Choi, N.K.; Kimura, M.; Kimura, T.; Kubota, K.; Lai, E.C.; Man, K.K.; Ooba, N.; Park, B.J.; et al. Prescription sequence symmetry analysis: Assessing risk, temporality, and consistency for adverse drug reactions across datasets in five countries. *Pharmacoepidemiol. Drug. Saf.* **2015**, *24*, 858–864. [CrossRef]
57. Roughead, E.E.; Chan, E.W.; Choi, N.K.; Kimura, M.; Kimura, T.; Kubota, K.; Lai, E.C.; Man, K.K.; Nguyen, T.A.; Ooba, N.; et al. Variation in Association Between Thiazolidinediones and Heart Failure Across Ethnic Groups: Retrospective analysis of Large Healthcare Claims Databases in Six Countries. *Drug Saf.* **2015**, *38*, 823–831. [CrossRef] [PubMed]
58. Roughead, E.E.; Chan, E.W.; Choi, N.K.; Griffiths, J.; Jin, X.M.; Lee, J.; Kimura, M.; Kimura, T.; Kubota, K.; Lai, E.C.; et al. Proton pump inhibitors and risk of Clostridium difficile infection: A multi-country study using sequence symmetry analysis. *Expert Opin. Drug Saf.* **2016**, *15*, 1589–1595. [CrossRef]
59. Man, K.K.C.; Shao, S.C.; Chaiyakunapruk, N.; Dilokthornsakul, P.; Kubota, K.; Li, J.; Ooba, N.; Pratt, N.; Pottegård, A.; Rasmussen, L.; et al. Metabolic events associated with the use of antipsychotics in children, adolescents and young adults: A multinational sequence symmetry study. *Eur. Child Adolesc. Psychiatry* **2020**. Online ahead of print. [CrossRef] [PubMed]

60. Hálfdánarson, Ó.; Zoëga, H.; Aagaard, L.; Bernardo, M.; Brandt, L.; Fusté, A.C.; Furu, K.; Garuolienė, K.; Hoffmann, F.; Huybrechts, K.F.; et al. International trends in antipsychotic use: A study in 16 countries, 2005–2014. *Eur. Neuropsychopharmacol.* **2017**, *27*, 1064–1076. [CrossRef] [PubMed]
61. Cohen, J.M.; Cesta, C.E.; Furu, K.; Einarsdóttir, K.; Gissler, M.; Havard, A.; Hernandez-Diaz, S.; Huybrechts, K.F.; Kieler, H.; Leinonen, M.K.; et al. Prevalence trends and individual patterns of antiepileptic drug use in pregnancy 2006–2016: A study in the five Nordic countries, United States, and Australia. *Pharmacoepidemiol. Drug. Saf.* **2020**, *29*, 913–922. [CrossRef] [PubMed]
62. Canadian Network for Observational Drug Effect Studies. CNODES Projects. Available online: https://www.cnodes.ca/projects/ (accessed on 25 August 2021).
63. Suissa, S.; Henry, D.; Caetano, P.; Dormuth, C.R.; Ernst, P.; Hemmelgarn, B.; Lelorier, J.; Levy, A.; Martens, P.J.; Paterson, J.M.; et al. CNODES: The Canadian Network for Observational Drug Effect Studies. *Open Med.* **2012**, *6*, e134–e140.
64. Platt, R.; Brown, J.S.; Robb, M.; McClellan, M.; Ball, R.; Nguyen, M.D.; Sherman, R.E. The FDA Sentinel Initiative—An Evolving National Resource. *N. Engl. J. Med.* **2018**, *379*, 2091–2093. [CrossRef]
65. Pormohammad, A.; Zarei, M.; Ghorbani, S.; Mohammadi, M.; Razizadeh, M.H.; Turner, D.L.; Turner, R.J. Efficacy and Safety of COVID-19 Vaccines: A Systematic Review and Meta-Analysis of Randomized Clinical Trials. *Vaccines* **2021**, *9*, 467. [CrossRef]
66. National COVID-19 Clinical Evidence Taskforce. Available online: https://covid19evidence.net.au/ (accessed on 13 September 2021).
67. Fosbøl, E.L.; Butt, J.H.; Østergaard, L.; Andersson, C.; Selmer, C.; Kragholm, K.; Schou, M.; Phelps, M.; Gislason, G.H.; Gerds, T.A.; et al. Association of Angiotensin-Converting Enzyme Inhibitor or Angiotensin Receptor Blocker Use with COVID-19 Diagnosis and Mortality. *JAMA* **2020**, *324*, 168–177. [CrossRef] [PubMed]
68. Dagan, N.; Barda, N.; Kepten, E.; Miron, O.; Perchik, S.; Katz, M.A.; Hernán, M.A.; Lipsitch, M.; Reis, B.; Balicer, R.D. BNT162b2 mRNA Covid-19 Vaccine in a Nationwide Mass Vaccination Setting. *N. Engl. J. Med.* **2021**, *384*, 1412–1423. [CrossRef]
69. Henry, D.A.; Jones, M.A.; Stehlik, P.; Glasziou, P.P. Effectiveness of COVID-19 vaccines: Findings from real world studies. *Med. J. Aust.* **2021**, *215*, 149–151.e141. [CrossRef]
70. NPS MedicineWise. *The Impact of COVID-19 on Hydroxychloroquine and Azithromycin Prescribing Patterns in General Practice*; NPS MedicineWise: Sydney, Australia, 2020.
71. Mian, M.; Sreedharan, S.; Giles, S. Increased dispensing of prescription medications in Australia early in the COVID-19 pandemic. *Med. J. Aust.* **2021**, *214*, 428–429. [CrossRef] [PubMed]
72. Engstrom, T.; Baliunas, D.O.; Sly, B.P.; Russell, A.W.; Donovan, P.J.; Krausse, H.K.; Sullivan, C.M.; Pole, J.D. Toilet Paper, Minced Meat and Diabetes Medicines: Australian Panic Buying Induced by COVID-19. *Int. J. Environ. Res. Public Health* **2021**, *18*, 6954. [CrossRef]
73. Kisely, S.; Dangelo-Kemp, D.; Taylor, M.; Liu, D.; Graham, S.; Hartmann, J.; Colman, S. The impact of COVID-19 on antipsychotic prescriptions for patients with schizophrenia in Australia. *Aust. N. Z. J. Psychiatry* **2021**. [CrossRef] [PubMed]
74. Tang, M.; Daniels, B.; Aslam, M.; Schaffer, A.; Pearson, S.A. Changes in systemic cancer therapy in Australia during the COVID-19 pandemic: A population-based study. *Lancet Reg. Health West Pac.* **2021**, *14*, 100226. [CrossRef]
75. Gillies, M.B.; Burgner, D.P.; Ivancic, L.; Nassar, N.; Miller, J.E.; Sullivan, S.G.; Todd, I.M.F.; Pearson, S.A.; Schaffer, A.L.; Zoega, H. Changes in antibiotic prescribing following COVID-19 restrictions: Lessons for post-pandemic antibiotic stewardship. *Br. J. Clin. Pharmacol.* **2021**. Online ahead of print. [CrossRef] [PubMed]
76. Lopez Bernal, J.; Andrews, N.; Gower, C.; Gallagher, E.; Simmons, R.; Thelwall, S.; Stowe, J.; Tessier, E.; Groves, N.; Dabrera, G.; et al. Effectiveness of Covid-19 Vaccines against the B.1.617.2 (Delta) Variant. *N. Engl. J. Med.* **2021**, *385*, 585–594. [CrossRef]
77. Hippisley-Cox, J.; Patone, M.; Mei, X.W.; Saatci, D.; Dixon, S.; Khunti, K.; Zaccardi, F.; Watkinson, P.; Shankar-Hari, M.; Doidge, J.; et al. Risk of thrombocytopenia and thromboembolism after covid-19 vaccination and SARS-CoV-2 positive testing: Self-controlled case series study. *BMJ* **2021**, *374*, n1931. [CrossRef]
78. Australian Institute of Health and Welfare. COVID-19: The Next Normal—Strengthening the System for 2021 and beyond. Available online: https://www.aihw.gov.au/reports-data/australias-health-performance/covid-19-the-next-normal-strengthening-the-system (accessed on 10 September 2021).
79. Scholl, H.J.; Patin, B.J.J. Resilient information infrastructures: Criticality and role in responding to catastrophic incidents. *Transform. Gov. People Process Policy* **2014**, *8*, 28–48. [CrossRef]
80. Productivity Commission. *Productivity Commission Inquiry Report: Data Availability and Use*; Australian Government: Canberra, Australia, 2017. Available online: https://www.pc.gov.au/inquiries/completed/data-access/report/data-access.pdf (accessed on 1 September 2021).
81. Senate Select Committee on Health. *Sixth Interim Report, Big Health Data: Australia's Big Potential*; Parliament of Australia: Canberra, Australia, 2016.
82. The National Cabinet. Intergovernmental Agreement on Data Sharing between Commonwealth and State and Territory Governments. Available online: https://federation.gov.au/about/agreements/intergovernmental-agreement-data-sharing (accessed on 24 August 2021).
83. Desai, T.; Ritchie, F.; Welpton, R. *Five Safes: Designing Data Access for Research*; University of the West of England: Bristol, UK, 2016.
84. The National Health and Medical Research Council: The Australian Research Council and Universities Australia. *National Statement on Ethical Conduct in Human Research 2007 (Updated 2018)*; Commonwealth of Australia: Canberra, Australia, 2018.

85. Briffa, T.G.; Jorm, L.; Jackson, R.T.; Reid, C.; Chew, D.P. Nationally linked data to improve health services and policy. *Med. J. Aust.* **2019**, *211*, 397–398.e391. [CrossRef]
86. Victorian Agency for Health Information. *Delivering Better Cardiac Outcomes in Victoria*; VAHI: Melbourne, Australia, 2019.
87. Falster, M.O.; Schaffer, A.L.; Wilson, A.; Nasis, A.; Jorm, L.R.; Hay, M.; Leeb, K.; Pearson, S.A.; Brieger, D. Evidence-practice gaps in P2Y(12) inhibitor use after hospitalisation for acute myocardial infarction: Findings from a new population-level data linkage in Australia. *Intern. Med. J.* **2020**. Online ahead of print. [CrossRef]
88. Schaffer, A.L.; Falster, M.O.; Brieger, D.; Jorm, L.R.; Wilson, A.; Hay, M.; Leeb, K.; Pearson, S.; Nasis, A. Evidence-Practice Gaps in Postdischarge Initiation With Oral Anticoagulants in Patients With Atrial Fibrillation. *J. Am. Heart Assoc.* **2019**, *8*, e014287. [CrossRef] [PubMed]
89. Schmidt, M.; Hallas, J.; Laursen, M.; Friis, S. Data Resource Profile: Danish online drug use statistics (MEDSTAT). *Int. J. Epidemiol.* **2016**, *45*, 1401–1402g. [CrossRef] [PubMed]
90. Solomon, M.D.; Majumdar, S.R. Primary non-adherence of medications: Lifting the veil on prescription-filling behaviors. *J. Gen. Intern. Med.* **2010**, *25*, 280–281. [CrossRef] [PubMed]
91. Whitehead, M.; Dahlgren, G. Concepts and principles for tackling social inequities in health: Levelling up Part 1. In *World Health Organization: Studies on Social and Economic Determinants of Population Health*; World Health Organization: Geneva, Switzerland, 2006; Volume 2, pp. 460–474.
92. Mourby, M.J.; Doidge, J.; Jones, K.H.; Aidinlis, S.; Smith, H.; Bell, J.; Gilbert, R.; Dutey-Magni, P.; Kaye, J. Health Data Linkage for UK Public Interest Research: Key Obstacles and Solutions. *Int. J. Popul. Data Sci.* **2019**, *4*, 1093. [CrossRef]
93. European Comission. European Health Data Space. Available online: https://ec.europa.eu/health/ehealth/dataspace_en (accessed on 13 September 2021).
94. Observational Health Data Sciences and Informatics. Chapter 4: OMOP Common Data Model. In *The Book of OHDSI*; OHDSI: New York, NY, USA, 2019.
95. Wang, S.V.; Schneeweiss, S.; Berger, M.L.; Brown, J.; de Vries, F.; Douglas, I.; Gagne, J.J.; Gini, R.; Klungel, O.; Mullins, C.D.; et al. Reporting to Improve Reproducibility and Facilitate Validity Assessment for Healthcare Database Studies V1.0. *Value Health* **2017**, *20*, 1009–1022. [CrossRef]
96. International Society for Pharmacoepidemiology (ISPE). RWE Task Force. Available online: https://www.pharmacoepi.org/strategic-initiatives/rwe-task-force/ (accessed on 30 August 2021).

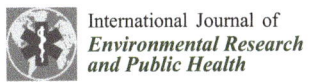

Article

Oral Health of Australian Adults: Distribution and Time Trends of Dental Caries, Periodontal Disease and Tooth Loss

Najith Amarasena *, Sergio Chrisopoulos, Lisa M. Jamieson and Liana Luzzi

Australian Research Centre for Population Oral Health (ARCPOH), Adelaide Dental School, Faculty of Medical and Health Sciences, The University of Adelaide, Adelaide 5000, Australia; sergio.chrisopoulos@adelaide.edu.au (S.C.); lisa.jamieson@adelaide.edu.au (L.M.J.); liana.luzzi@adelaide.edu.au (L.L.)
* Correspondence: najith.amarasena@adelaide.edu.au

Citation: Amarasena, N.; Chrisopoulos, S.; Jamieson, L.M.; Luzzi, L. Oral Health of Australian Adults: Distribution and Time Trends of Dental Caries, Periodontal Disease and Tooth Loss. *Int. J. Environ. Res. Public Health* **2021**, *18*, 11539. https://doi.org/10.3390/ijerph182111539

Academic Editor: Paul B. Tchounwou

Received: 15 September 2021
Accepted: 28 October 2021
Published: 2 November 2021

Publisher's Note: MDPI stays neutral with regard to jurisdictional claims in published maps and institutional affiliations.

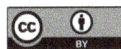

Copyright: © 2021 by the authors. Licensee MDPI, Basel, Switzerland. This article is an open access article distributed under the terms and conditions of the Creative Commons Attribution (CC BY) license (https://creativecommons.org/licenses/by/4.0/).

Abstract: This study was conducted to describe the distribution and trends in dental caries, periodontal disease and tooth loss in Australian adults based on the findings of the National Study of Adult Oral Health 2017–18. A cross-sectional study of a random sample of Australians aged 15+ years was carried out, employing a three-stage stratified probability sampling design. Data were collected via online survey/telephone interviews using a questionnaire to elicit self-reported information about oral health and related characteristics. Participants were then invited to have an oral examination, conducted by calibrated dental practitioners following a standardised protocol in public dental clinics. A total of 15,731 Australians aged 15+ years were interviewed, of which 5022 dentate participants were orally examined. Results showed that nearly one third of Australian adults had at least one tooth surface with untreated dental caries and, on average, 29.7 decayed, missing or filled tooth surfaces per person. Almost 29% of adults presented with gingivitis while the overall prevalence of periodontitis was 30.1%. Overall, 4% of adults were edentulous while, on average, 4.4 teeth were lost due to pathology. Poorer oral health was evident in Australians from lower socioeconomic backgrounds, indicating socioeconomic inequalities in oral health. Time trends revealed that dental caries experience and tooth retention of Australian adults has improved over 30 years, while periodontal health has deteriorated between 2004–06 and 2017–18. These findings can be used to assist policy makers in planning and implementing future oral healthcare programs.

Keywords: dental caries; oral health; periodontal disease; tooth loss

1. Introduction

Traditionally, oral health has been defined as "a state of being free from mouth and facial pain, oral diseases and disorders that limit an individual's capacity in biting, chewing, smiling, speaking and psychosocial well-being" [1]. In view of more emphasis given to 'absence of disease' in this definition, a broader description for oral health has recently been suggested [2]. This broader definition advocates the definitions adopted by global and national organizations and reiterates the importance of recognising dentistry as an arena providing care and supporting oral health, rather than purely treating disease. According to the new definition, oral health is multi-faceted and includes the ability to speak, smile, smell, taste, touch, chew, swallow and convey a range of emotions through facial expressions with confidence and without pain, discomfort, and disease of the craniofacial complex, as well as being a fundamental component of general health and physical and mental wellbeing [2,3]. While proponents of this new definition aimed to reach consensus on a universal definition of oral health, this has not eventuated [4]. Global oral health aims to provide optimal oral health for all and to eradicate global health inequalities via health promotion, disease prevention and appropriate oral care strategies that incorporate common factors and resolutions, and recognise that oral health is integral to overall health [4].

Oral diseases predominantly comprise tooth decay (dental caries), gingival (periodontal) disease and oral cancers [5,6]. Dental caries, which is considered the most prevalent chronic disease worldwide [7], occur when microorganisms of dental biofilm (a sticky colourless film of bacteria build-up on the tooth surfaces) start to metabolize fermentable carbohydrates in the diet, in particular, free sugars, into acidic by-products. These acidic by-products can locally destroy (demineralise) the hard tooth structure (enamel and dentine) and initiate dental caries' development. Frequent consumption of high free sugar and insufficient exposure to fluoride are the main contributing factors for dental caries [5–7]. While making enamel more resistant to acid attack, fluoride mainly acts topically to inhibit demineralisation through its presence at low concentrations in the oral fluids [5,7]. With periodontal disease, tissues that support and surround the tooth (gums, periodontal ligament and alveolar bone) are affected mainly by dental biofilm accumulated at the neck of the tooth where the tissues meet the gums (gingival margin), causing gingivitis (bleeding of the gums) [5,6]. This may lead to a more destructive form of disease, i.e., periodontitis, in susceptible individuals, particularly among those who are immunocompromised [5,6]. Poor oral hygiene, accompanied by inadequate plaque removal, is the main cause of periodontal disease, while tobacco smoking is a major risk factor associated with periodontal disease [5,6]. If left untreated, both dental caries and periodontal disease lead to tooth loss, and these two oral diseases are the major causes of tooth loss. Oral diseases affect nearly 3.5 billion people universally. Of them, approximately 2.3 billion and 530 million present with dental caries of the permanent and primary (baby) dentitions, respectively [8,9]. In 2010, severe periodontitis was ranked as the sixth-most prevalent health condition, afflicting 743 million people globally with an incidence of 701 cases per 100,000 person years [10]. Although the prevalence of severe tooth loss declined from 4.4% in 1990 to 2.4% in 2010, 158 million people worldwide were edentulous in 2010 [10].

In regard to the oral health status of Australians (based on data published prior to the National Study of Adult Oral Health 2017–18), 42% and 24% of children aged 5–10 years and 6–14 years, respectively, had experienced dental caries in their primary teeth and permanent teeth, whereas almost a quarter of Australian dentate adults aged 15 and over had untreated decay [11]. The prevalence of periodontal disease in Australian dentate adults aged 15 years and over was 22.9%, whilst 4.4% of the adult population were edentulous [11]. The present study aims at describing the distribution and time trends of dental caries, periodontal disease and tooth loss in Australian adults based on findings from the National Study of Adult Oral Health 2017–18 (NSAOH 2017–18).

2. Materials & Methods

Study methodology, including computation of sample size, has been described in previous studies [12,13]. Briefly, a cross-sectional study of a random sample of Australians aged 15 years and over was carried out across all Australian states and territories, employing a three-stage stratified probability sampling design. The first stage of selection included sampling of postcodes within states/territories, mainly by means of systematic sampling with probability of selection proportional to the number of households within the postcode, followed by selecting individuals aged 15 years and over within selected postcodes from the Medicare database provided by the Australian Government Department of Human Services (DHS). Accordingly, the final sample size required 15,200 interviews to be conducted, in order to complete 7200 oral examinations.

Interviews were conducted online or by telephone (CATI—computer-assisted telephone interview) by trained interviewers using a questionnaire based on previous surveys [11,14]. Self-reported information about oral health and related characteristics such as age, sex, Indigenous identity, residential location, schooling/educational qualifications, eligibility for public dental care, dental insurance and usual reason for a visit to the dentist was collected. Calibrated dental practitioners conducted oral examinations following a standardised protocol in public dental clinics run by the relevant state or territory dental health services. Inter-examiner reliability relative to a gold standard examiner was assessed by conducting replicate pairs of examination with 101 study participants. Dentate participants who consented to an examination were included for oral examinations. Although there were nine measures of oral health status, as described in detail elsewhere [15], the current analysis was confined to assessment of coronal caries (dental decay in tooth crown), gingivitis and periodontal destruction, and presence/absence of teeth (tooth loss).

2.1. Dental Caries (Coronal Caries)

All teeth present were subdivided into five tooth surfaces and assessed for dental caries using visual criteria without an explorer. The five tooth surfaces were mesial, buccal, distal, lingual and occlusal (for back teeth: premolars and molars)/incisal (for front teeth: incisors and canines). The mean number of decayed tooth surfaces per person denotes the severity, or burden, of untreated dental caries in people. The number of decayed, missing and filled tooth surfaces (DMFS) indicates lifetime experience of dental caries in a given person, since it has been regarded that cavities in enamel cannot heal and treatment of dental decay, either as a filling or extraction, leaves a permanent sign of disease [12].

2.2. Periodontal Disease

Clinical assessment for periodontal disease was conducted among those who had no medical contraindications for periodontal probing. Gingivitis and periodontitis were the two types of diseases assessed, as per the following criteria:

Gingivitis: Inflammation of the marginal gingival tissues around six index teeth (if present: the most anterior molar tooth in each dental quadrant + right upper central incisor + left lower central incisor) were assessed using the gingival index of Loe and Silness [16].

Periodontitis: The US National Health and Nutrition Examination Survey (NHANES) methods were employed to assess periodontal tissue destruction [17]. Assessments were made on three aspects (mesio-buccal, mid-buccal and disto-buccal) of all teeth present, except third molars (wisdom teeth), using a periodontal probe. To describe the prevalence of moderate and severe periodontitis, a case definition developed by the US Centers for Disease Control and Prevention (CDC) and the American Academy of Periodontology (AAP) was used [17]. Accordingly, moderate periodontitis was defined as the presence of either at least two proximal sites not on the same tooth with attachment loss of 4 mm or more, or at least two such sites that had pockets of 5 mm or more. Severe periodontitis was defined as having at least two proximal sites not on the same tooth with attachment loss of 6 mm or more, plus at least one periodontal pocket with a depth of 5 mm or more.

Tooth loss: Complete tooth loss (edentulism) was assessed based on the answer to the following interview question: 'Do you have any natural teeth?', with response categories of 'Yes'/'No'. Existing natural teeth included crowns and caps, while dental implants were not considered natural teeth. For participants aged less than 45 years, the examiners distinguished between missing teeth that had been removed due to dental decay or periodontal disease and teeth missing due to any other reason. For participants aged 45 years or more, a removed or an absent tooth was recorded as missing.

To ensure representativeness of the target population, all data were weighted to population benchmarks [13]. Data files were managed and summary variables were computed using SAS software version 9.4 (SAS 9.4; SAS Institute Inc., Cary, NC, USA). Proportions, means and their 95% confidence were calculated where relevant.

3. Results

A total of 15,731 Australians aged 15 years and over completed an interview, and of them, 5022 dentate participants were orally examined. This resulted in overall participation rates of 39.7% (interview) and 33.6% (examination). Intra-class correlation coefficients (ICC) calculated to assess inter-examiner reliability were above 0.9 and 0.7 for diagnosing dental caries and periodontal disease, respectively. Weighting ensured that, approximately, an equal proportion of males (49.2%) and females (50.8) participated in the study. Given that oral health status varies considerably with age, population estimates were calculated for four age groups—15–34 years, 35–54 years, 55–74 years and ≥75 years. Tables 1–7 present the distribution of dental caries, periodontal disease and tooth loss, and Figures 1–3 depict the time trends of these three conditions.

Table 1. Proportion of Australian dentate adults aged 15 years and over with untreated coronal caries.

	N	% (95% CI)	Total	15–34	Age (Years) 35–54 % (95% CI)	55–74	≥75
All people	5022		32.1 (29.6, 34.7)	30.3 (25.7, 35.2)	35.4 (31.1, 40.0)	32.2 (28.2, 36.6)	24.5 (18.8, 31.3)
Sex							
Male	2249	49.6 (46.9, 52.2)	34.7 (31.2, 38.4)	32.1 (25.1, 40.0)	37.1 (30.9, 43.7)	38.5 (33.2, 44.2)	22.3 (14.8, 32.2)
Female	2773	50.4 (47.8, 53.1)	29.5 (26.3, 32.9)	28.4 (23.2, 24.2)	33.8 (28.3, 39.8)	26.0 (20.3, 32.6)	26.2 (18.3, 36.0)
Indigenous identity							
Non-Indigenous	4937	98.3 (97.4, 98.9)	32.1 (29.5, 34.7)	30.6 (26.0, 35.6)	35.4 (31.1, 40.0)	31.6 (27.6, 35.9)	24.5 (18.8, 31.3)
Indigenous	84	1.7 (1.1, 2.6)	* 27.8 (15.0, 45.5)	* 17.6 (6.8, 38.3)	* 36.1(15.5, 63.4)	72.8 (45.1, 89.7)	* 22.4 (2.6, 75.9)
Residential location							
Major cities	2969	72.7 (69.1, 76.0)	31.8 (28.7, 35.1)	28.0 (23.4, 33.2)	35.3 (29.9, 41.2)	34.9 (29.4, 40.7)	25.7 (18.2, 34.9)
Rural/remote	2053	27.3 (24.0, 30.9)	32.6 (28.4, 37.1)	35.9 (26.0, 47.1)	35.6 (29.3, 42.6)	28.0 (22.4, 34.4)	22.5 (14.9, 32.5)
Year level of schooling							
Year 10 or less	1190	25.5 (23.5, 27.8)	36.9 (32.0, 42.1)	32.8 (22.4, 45.3)	51.4 (41.1, 61.6)	35.0 (28.0, 42.7)	25.3 (17.7, 34.7)
Year 11 or more	3793	74.5 (72.2, 76.5)	30.2 (27.3, 33.2)	29.6 (25.0, 34.7)	31.7 (27.1, 36.8)	29.7 (25.1, 34.9)	22.5 (14.3, 33.7)
Highest qualification attained							
Degree or higher	2026	29.3 (26.9, 31.8)	30.4 (26.3, 34.8)	33.1 (26.4, 40.4)	29.3 (23.6, 35.7)	27.6 (21.4, 34.7)	* 14.5 (7.7, 25.5)
Other/None	2931	70.7 (68.2, 73.1)	32.6 (29.5, 35.8)	28.6 (22.9, 35.0)	39.0 (33.2, 45.1)	32.6 (27.9, 37.6)	24.9 (18.7, 32.3)
Eligibility for public dental care							
Eligible	1634	30.7 (28.3, 33.1)	34.5 (30.1, 39.1)	29.3 (18.8, 42.6)	54.2 (45.5, 62.7)	32.9 (26.6, 39.8)	24.1 (18.1, 31.5)
Ineligible	3373	69.3 (66.9, 71.7)	31.1 (28.1, 34.2)	30.8 (26.0, 36.0)	31.4 (26.9, 36.3)	31.4 (26.3, 37.0)	* 26.7 (13.8, 45.4)
Dental insurance							
Insured	2548	45.3 (42.5, 48.1)	24.4 (21.3, 27.7)	22.3 (17.3, 28.4)	25.1 (19.8, 31.3)	25.9 (21.3, 31.1)	24.9 (17.0, 34.8)
Uninsured	2385	54.7 (51.9, 57.5)	38.6 (35.2, 42.1)	35.9 (29.8, 42.5)	45.7 (39.9, 51.6)	37.8 (31.5, 44.5)	24.3 (16.3, 34.6)
Usually visit dentist							
For a check-up	3135	61.5 (58.8, 64.1)	24.3 (21.4, 27.5)	24.2 (19.3, 29.9)	25.4 (20.3, 31.3)	24.4 (19.6, 30.0)	19.5 (13.1, 28.0)
For a dental problem	1796	38.5 (35.9, 41.2)	43.5 (39.3, 47.9)	43.7 (35.6, 52.2)	49.2 (42.5, 56.0)	39.4 (32.5, 46.7)	30.9 (20.1, 44.3)

* Indicates a relative standard error of at least 25%, and hence should be interpreted with caution.

Table 2. Mean number of decayed tooth surfaces per person in the Australian dentate adults aged 15 years and over.

	N	% (95% CI)	Total	15–34	Age (Years) 35–54 Mean (95% CI)	55–74	≥75
All people	5022		1.4 (1.2, 1.6)	1.3 (0.9, 1.7)	1.4 (1.1, 1.7)	1.8 (1.3, 2.3)	1.1 (0.6, 1.5)
Sex							
Male	2249	49.6 (46.9, 52.2)	1.7 (1.4, 2.0)	1.3 (0.8, 1.7)	1.6 (1.1, 2.1)	2.8 (1.9, 3.6)	1.1 * (0.3, 1.9)
Female	2773	50.4 (47.8, 53.1)	1.2 (0.9, 1.4)	1.4 (0.8, 1.9)	1.3 (0.9, 1.7)	0.8 (0.5, 1.0)	1.1 (0.6, 1.6)
Indigenous identity							
Non-Indigenous	4937	98.3 (97.4, 98.9)	1.4 (1.2, 1.6)	1.3 (0.9, 1.6)	1.4 (1.1, 1.7)	1.8 (1.3, 2.2)	1.1 (0.6, 1.6)
Indigenous	84	1.7 (1.1, 2.6)	2.7 * (0.5, 4.9)	2.5 * (0.0, 5.7)	3.2 * (0.2, 6.3)	2.8 * (0.0, 6.5)	0.9 * (0.0, 2.6)
Residential location							
Major cities	2969	72.7 (69.1, 76.0)	1.4 (1.1,1.6)	1.3 (0.8,1.7)	1.4 (1.0,1.8)	1.6 (1.0,2.1)	1.3 (0.6,1.9)
Rural/remote	2053	27.3 (24.0,30.9)	1.6 (1.3,2.0)	1.4 (0.9,1.9)	1.5 (1.1,2.0)	2.2 (1.3,3.2)	0.7 (0.4,1.0)
Year level of schooling							
Year 10 or less	1190	25.5 (23.5,27.8)	2.1 (1.6,2.6)	2.6 * (1.0,4.2)	2.2 (1.5,2.9)	2.2 (1.4,3.0)	1.3 * (0.6,2.0)
Year 11 or more	3793	74.5 (72.2,76.5)	1.2 (1.0,1.4)	1.1 (0.8,1.4)	1.3 (0.9,1.6)	1.3 (0.9,1.6)	0.7 (0.4,1.0)
Highest qualification attained							
Degree or above	2026	29.3 (26.9,31.8)	0.9 (0.7,1.2)	0.9 (0.6,1.3)	0.9 (0.5,1.2)	1.1 (0.6,1.7)	0.9 * (0.2,1.7)
Other/None	2931	70.7 (68.2,73.1)	1.7 (1.4,1.9)	1.5 (0.9,2.1)	1.7 (1.3,2.2)	2 (1.4,2.5)	1.1 (0.5,1.6)
Eligibility for public dental care							
Eligible	1634	30.7 (28.3,33.1)	2.1 (1.6,2.5)	1.8 * (0.6,3.0)	2.9 (2.1,3.8)	2.3 (1.4,3.1)	1.1 (0.6,1.7)
Ineligible	3373	69.3 (66.9,71.7)	1.2 (1.0,1.4)	1.2 (0.8,1.5)	1.1 (0.8,1.4)	1.3 (0.9,1.8)	0.8 * (0.3,1.3)
Dental insurance							
Insured	2548	45.3 (42.5,48.1)	0.8 (0.6,1.0)	0.7 (0.4,0.9)	0.8 (0.5,1.1)	1.1 (0.7,1.6)	0.6 (0.4,0.9)
Uninsured	2385	54.7 (51.9,57.5)	1.9 (1.6,2.2)	1.6 (1.1,2.1)	2 (1.6,2.5)	2.3 (1.6,3.1)	1.4 * (0.6,2.3)
Usually visit dentist							
For a check-up	3135	61.5 (58.8,64.1)	0.7 (0.6,0.9)	0.7 (0.5,0.9)	0.8 (0.5,1.2)	0.6 (0.5,0.8)	0.5 (0.3,0.7)
For a dental problem	1796	38.5 (35.9,41.2)	2.3 (1.9,2.6)	2.4 (1.5,3.3)	2.1 (1.7,2.6)	2.4 (1.7,3.2)	1.8 * (0.7,2.9)

* Indicates a relative standard error of at least 25%, and hence should be interpreted with caution.

Table 3. Mean number of decayed, missing or filled tooth surfaces per person in Australian dentate adults aged 15 years and over.

	N	Weighted %	Total	15–34	Age (Years) 35–54 Mean (95% CI)	55–74	≥75
All people	5022		29.7 (28.4, 31.1)	7.7 (6.9, 8.5)	24.9 (23.3, 26.5)	57.1 (54.8, 59.4)	75.3 (72.2, 78.4)
Sex							
Male	2249	49.6 (46.9,52.2)	27.1 (25.2, 29.1)	7.3 (6.0, 8.5)	22.2 (19.8, 24.5)	53.5 (50.5, 56.4)	71.5 67.1, 76.0)
Female	2773	50.4 (47.8,53.1)	32.3 (30.5, 34.1)	8.1 (6.9, 9.4)	27.6 (25.6, 29.6)	60.7 (57.3, 64.2)	78.3 (74.5, 82.1)
Indigenous identity							
Non-Indigenous	4937	98.3 (97.4,98.9)	29.9 (28.5, 31.3)	7.7 (6.9, 8.6)	24.9 (23.3, 26.5)	57.1 (54.8, 59.5)	75.4 (72.3, 78.5)
Indigenous	84	1.7 (1.1,2.6)	18.7 (10.3, 27.1)	* 6.9 (1.1, 12.7)	27.5 (22.7, 32.3)	63.9 (54.9, 72.8)	NP
Residential location							
Major cities	2969	72.7 (69.1,76.0)	28.5 (26.9, 30.1)	7.8 (6.8, 8.9)	24.4 (22.5, 26.3)	57 (53.6, 60.4)	77.8 (73.8, 81.7)
Rural/remote	2053	27.3 (24.0,30.9)	32.3 (29.8, 34.8)	7.3 (5.9, 8.8)	26 (23.1, 28.9)	57.2 (54.7, 59.7)	71.1 (66.9, 75.4)
Year level of schooling							
Year 10 or less	1190	25.5 (23.5,27.8)	43.9 (41.1–46.8)	7.6 (4.6, 10.6)	29.9 (26.1, 33.8)	57 (53.4, 60.7)	75.6 (71.2, 80.0)
Year 11 or more	3793	74.5 (72.2,76.5)	24.8 (23.4, 26.2)	7.6 (6.8, 8.5)	23.9 (22.1, 25.6)	57.3 (54.3, 60.3)	74.8 (71.2, 78.4)
Highest qualification attained							
Degree or higher	2026	29.3 (26.9,31.8)	20.9 (19.2, 22.5)	8.4 (7.2, 9.6)	19 (17.1, 20.8)	55.8 (52.9, 58.7)	76.3 (72.0, 80.6)
Other/None	2931	70.7 (68.2,73.1)	33.4 (31.8, 35.1)	7.3 (6.2, 8.4)	28.3 (26.1, 30.5)	58 (55.4, 60.5)	75.7 (72.1, 79.2)
Eligibility for public dental care							
Eligible	1634	30.7 (28.3,33,1)	44.8 (42.0, 47.6)	8.8 (6.8, 10.7)	32.5 (28.6, 36.4)	58.9 (55.2, 62.5)	75.5 (72.0–79.0)
Ineligible	3373	69.3 (66.9,71.7)	23.2 (21.8, 24.5)	7.5 (6.6, 8.4)	23.3 (21.6, 25.0)	55.4 (52.5, 58.3)	74.1 (69.2, 79.0)
Dental insurance							
Insured	2548	45.3 (42.5,48,1)	30.6 (28.8, 32.4)	7.5 (6.2, 8.7)	23.2 (21.1, 25.4)	59.4 (57.0, 61.8)	76.4 (72.8, 79.9)
Uninsured	2385	54.7 (51.9,57.5)	29.9 (27.9, 31.8)	7.9 (6.8, 9.1)	27.1 (24.6, 29.5)	55.3 (51.6, 59.0)	74.6 (69.8, 79.3)
Usually visit dentist							
For a check-up	3135	61.5 (58.8,64,1)	26.6 (25.0, 28.1)	6.5 (5.6, 7.3)	21.9 (19.8, 23.9)	56.7 (54.3, 59.2)	75.5 (71.1, 79.8)
For a dental problem	1796	38.5 (35.9,41.2)	35.7 (33.4, 37.9)	10.8 (8.9, 12.7)	29.8 (27.2, 32.4)	57.7 (53.5, 61.9)	75.3 (71.1, 79.4)

* Indicates a relative standard error of at least 25%, and hence should be interpreted with caution. NP: Not publishable due to small cell counts.

Table 4. Percentage of people with gingival inflammation in the Australian dentate population.

	N	% (95% CI)	Total	15–34	Age (Years) 35–54 % (95% CI)	55–74	≥75
All people	4401		28.8 (26.1, 31.6)	31.3 (27.1, 35.8)	29.5 (25.2, 34.2)	24.4 (20.7, 28.6)	20.9 (15.0, 28.2)
Sex							
Male	1906	48.9 (46.0,51.8)	34.7 (30.7,39.0)	34.9 (28.5,41.8)	35.6 (29.3,42.4)	34.1 (28.0,40.8)	27.4 (17.0,41.1)
Female	2496	51.1 (48.2,54.0)	23.1 (20.3,26.1)	27.6 (22.7,33.0)	23.7 (18.8,29.3)	15.7 (12.1,20.3)	16.7 (10.3,26.0)
Indigenous identity							
Non-Indigenous	4330	98.4 (97.4,99.0)	28.7 (26.0,31.5)	31.3 (27.0,35.9)	29.1 (24.8,33.8)	24.6 (20.8,28.9)	20.9 (15.1,28.2)
Indigenous	71	1.6 (1.0,2.6)	38.6 (19.9,61.4)	30.5 * (11.1,60.7)	63.3 (36.2,84.0)	9.9 * (1.2,49.2)	NP
Residential location							
Major cities	2607	73.8 (70.3,77.0)	30.1 (26.8,33.5)	31.5 (26.8,36.6)	31.6 (26.2,37.5)	26.0 (21.0,31.7)	21.9 (14.9,30.8)
Rural/remote	1795	26.2 (23.0,29.7)	25.2 (20.6,30.4)	30.4 (21.8,40.6)	24.2 (18.1,31.4)	21.1 (16.3,26.9)	18.2 * (9.2,32.9)
Year level of schooling							
Year 10 or less	943	23.2 (21.2,25.4)	28.6 (24.0,33.8)	40.2 (27.5,54.3)	30.4 (22.1,40.1)	23.3 (17.5,30.2)	18.6 (11.4,28.8)
Year 11 or more	3427	76.8 (74.6,78.8)	28.9 (25.9,32.1)	29.9 (25.5,34.7)	29.3 (24.6,34.6)	25.6 (21.0,30.9)	24.5 (15.7,36.0)
Highest qualification attained							
Degree or above	1865	30.6 (28.1,33.3)	24.0 (20.5,28.0)	21.3 v	27.3 (21.2,34.3)	24.2 (17.5,32.5)	22.2 * (11.3,39.1)
Other/None	2477	69.4 (66.7,71.9)	31.2 (27.9,34.6)	36.7 (31.1,42.7)	31.0 (25.6,37.0)	25.2 (20.9,30.0)	20.7 (14.1,29.3)
Eligibility for public dental care							
Eligible	1264	27.3 (24.9,29.9)	30.4 (26.0,35.3)	31.9 (22.8,42.5)	38.1 (29.1,48.0)	28.4 (22.2,35.5)	19.6 (13.5,27.6)
Ineligible	3123	72.7 (70.1,75.1)	28.3 (25.3,31.5)	31.3 (26.7,36.4)	27.8 (23.3,32.8)	21.4 (17.0,26.4)	29.6 * (14.1,51.8)
Dental insurance							
Insured	2261	46.1 (43.0,49.2)	25.2 (22.0,28.8)	29.9 (24.0,36.5)	25.0 (19.8,31.1)	20.4 (16.2,25.3)	14.9 (9.1,23.6)
Uninsured	2058	53.9 (50.8,57.0)	31.1 (27.5,34.9)	30.1 (24.6,36.1)	34.8 (28.6,41.6)	28.4 (22.5,35.1)	25.8 (16.9,37.3)
Usually visit dentist							
For a check-up	2775	62.3 (59.5,65.1)	25.2 (22.0,28.7)	27.5 (22.5,33.1)	25.2 (20.2,31.1)	20.7 (16.7,25.3)	20.5 (13.6,29.9)
For a dental problem	1548	37.7 (34.9,40.5)	33.2 (29.3,37.4)	35.4 (27.9,43.6)	35.7 (29.3,42.8)	28.7 (22.6,35.8)	21.4 * (12.2,34.9)

* Indicates a relative standard error of at least 25%, and hence should be interpreted with caution. NP: not publishable due to small cell counts.

Table 5. Proportion of people with moderate or severe periodontitis in the Australian dentate population.

	N	% (95% CI)	Total	15–34	Age (Years) 35–54 % (95% CI)	55–74	≥75
All people	4402		30.1 (27.9, 32.4)	12.2 (9.5, 15.6)	32.7 (28.5, 37.3)	51.1 (46.2, 56.0)	69.3 (60.5, 76.9)
Sex							
Male	1906	48.9 (46.0,51.8)	34.9 (31.2,38.8)	16.6 (11.8,22.8)	38.9 (32.1,46.3)	59.5 (53.3,65.4)	63.1 (48.1,75.9)
Female	2496	51.1 (48.2,54.0)	25.5 (22.7,28.5)	7.8 (5.3,11.3)	26.6 (21.7,32.2)	43.5 (37.1,50.2)	73.0 (62.3,81.6)
Indigenous identity							
Non-Indigenous	4330	98.4 (97.4,99.0)	30.3 (28.1,32.7)	12.5 (9.7,15.9)	32.9 (28.6,37.5)	50.8 (46.0,55.6)	69.2 (60.4,76.8)
Indigenous	71	1.6 (1.0,2.6)	11.0 * (5.3,21.3)	3.9 * (0.8,17.2)	21.0 * (8.2,44.1)	49.7 * (15.4,84.3)	NP
Residential location							
Major cities	2607	73.8(70.3,77.0)	29.4 (26.7,32.2)	12.2 (9.0,16.4)	31.6 (26.4,37.2)	52.9 (46.7,59.1)	71.1 (60.1,80.0)
Rural/remote	1795	26.2 (23.0,29.7)	32.1 (28.1,36.5)	12.3 (8.2,18.2)	35.8 (28.8,43.4)	47.1 (39.6,54.8)	64.4 (49.7,76.9)
Year level of schooling							
Year 10 or less	943	23.2 (21.2,25.4)	45.0 (39.6,50.5)	7.7 * (3.3,16.7)	50.0 (39.8,60.3)	55.9 (47.8,63.7)	72.2 (61.0,81.1)
Year 11 or more	3427	76.8 (74.6,78.8)	25.6 (23.2,28.2)	12.9 (9.8,16.8)	29.2 (24.8,34.1)	47.8 (42.3,53.3)	64.7 (49.2,77.7)
Highest qualification attained							
Degree or above	1865	23.2 (21.2,25.4)	21.7 (18.2,25.6)	11.6 (6.7,19.1)	22.7 (18.1,28.1)	49.7 (42.6,56.7)	59.6 (35.9,79.6)
Other/None	2477	69.4 (66.7,71.9)	33.6 (30.6,36.6)	12.6 (9.5,16.5)	38.4 (32.5,44.6)	50.9 (45.3,56.5)	69.9 (60.6,77.8)
Eligibility for public dental care							
Eligible	1264	27.3 (24.9,29.9)	42.5 (37.9,47.2)	15.7 (9.0,25.9)	41.3 (32.1,51.2)	54.8 (47.5,61.9)	70.6 (61.5,78.3)
Ineligible	3123	72.7 (70.1,75.1)	25.5 (22.9,28.2)	11.5 (8.7,14.9)	30.9 (26.2,36.0)	47.7 (41.8,53.7)	59.3 (33.3,80.9)
Dental insurance							
Insured	2261	46.1 (43.0,49.2)	25.4 (22.7,28.3)	8.4 (5.1,13.4)	24.5 (19.8,30.0)	45.2 (39.0,51.6)	67.4 (53.1,79.1)
Uninsured	2058	53.9 (50.8,57.0)	35.0 (31.8,38.4)	15.7 (11.5,20.9)	41.1 (34.8,47.7)	56.9 (49.7,63.8)	70.7 (59.7,79.8)
Usually visit dentist							
For a check-up	2775	62.3 (59.5,65.1)	26.1 (23.4,29.0)	8.8 (6.0,12.9)	29.5 (23.9,35.8)	49.0 (43.0,55.0)	72.5 (60.4,81.9)
For a dental problem	1548	37.7 (34.9,40.5)	36.8 (32.6,41.3)	18.8 (13.4,25.8)	37.2 (30.4,44.5)	53.0 (45.6,60.2)	64.3 (50.3,76.2)

* Indicates a relative standard error of at least 25%, and hence should be interpreted with caution. NP: not publishable due to small cell counts.

Table 6. Proportion of adults with complete tooth loss in the Australian population.

	N	% (95% CI)	Total	15–34	Age (Years) 35–54 % (95% CI)	55–74	≥75
All people	15,731		4.0 (3.6, 4.4)	—	1.1 (0.7, 1.6)	8.1 (7.0, 9.3)	20.5 (18.1, 23.1)
Sex							
Male	6781	49.2 (48.1,50.4)	3.4 (2.9,3.9)	—	1.1 * (0.6,2.0)	6.5 (5.2,8.1)	19.1 (15.6,23.2)
Female	8950	50.8 (49.6,51.9)	4.7 (4.1,5.3)	—	1.0 * (0.6,1.8)	9.6 (8.0,11.5)	21.5 (18.4,25.0)
Indigenous identity							
Non-Indigenous	15,392	97.7 (97.3,98.1)	4.0 (3.6,4.4)	—	1.1 (0.7,1.6)	7.7 (6.7,8.9)	20.5 (18.1,23.1)
Indigenous	334	2.3 (1.9,2.7)	7.1 (4.3,11.4)	—	0.8 * (0.2,2.5)	29.3 (17.8,44.1)	19.5 * (6.5,45.9)
Residential location							
Major cities	9372	71.8 (68.6,74.9)	3.5 (3.0,4.0)	—	1.0 * (0.6,1.7)	7.4 (6.0,9.0)	18.8 (15.9,22.0)
Rural/remote	6359	28.2 (25.1,31.4)	5.4 (4.7,6.2)	—	1.2 * (0.7,2.0)	9.5 (8.1,11.2)	24.2 (20.1,28.7)
Year level of schooling							
Year 10 or less	4198	28.9 (27.8,30.1)	9.4 (8.5,10.5)	—	3.1 * (1.8,5.2)	11.7 (9.9,13.8)	24.9 (21.6,28.5)
Year 11 or more	11,355	71.1 (69.9,72.2)	1.8 (1.5,2.1)	—	0.6 * (0.3,1.1)	5.3 (4.2,6.7)	13.1 (10.2,16.6)
Highest qualification attained							
Degree or higher	5836	26.8 (25.4,28.2)	0.7 (0.5,1.1)	—	0.5 * (0.1,1.6)	2.0 (1.3,3.1)	5.3 * (3.0,9.0)
Other/None	9584	73.2 (71.8,74.6)	5.1 (4.6,5.7)	—	1.3 (0.8,2.0)	9.4 (8.1,10.8)	22.0 (19.4,24.9)
Eligibility for public dental care							
Eligible	4976	30.2 (29.0,31.4)	10.5 (9.5,11.7)	—	3.1 * (1.7,5.3)	13.4 (11.5,15.6)	22.3 (19.6,25.2)
Ineligible	10,686	69.8 (68.6,71.0)	1.2 (1.0,1.5)	—	0.7 * (0.4,1.2)	3.7 (2.9,4.9)	11.3 (7.6,16.5)
Dental insurance							
Insured	8238	51.1 (49.5,52.8)	1.7 (1.4,2.0)	—	0.5 * (0.3,1.1)	3.6 (2.8,4.5)	9.2 (7.0,11.9)
Uninsured	7206	48.9 (47.2,50.5)	6.5 (5.8,7.2)	—	1.8 (1.1,2.8)	12.7 (10.9,14.8)	28.3 (24.7,32.3)
Usually visit dentist							
For a check-up	9790	63.3 (61.9,64.6)	1.2 (0.9,1.5)	—	0.3 * (0.2,0.6)	3.0 (2.1,4.2)	6.1 (4.4,8.4)
For a dental problem	5620	36.7 (35.4,38.1)	7.9 (7.1,8.8)	—	2.2 (1.3,3.5)	13.0 (11.2,15.0)	32.5 (28.5,36.7)

* Indicates a relative standard error of at least 25%, and hence should be interpreted with caution.

Table 7. Mean number of missing teeth for pathology per person in the Australian dentate population.

	N	% (95% CI)	Total	15–34	Age (Years) 35–54 Mean (95% CI)	55–74	≥75
All people	5022		4.4 (4.1, 4.7)	0.6 (0.4, 0.7)	3.6 (3.3, 3.9)	8.8 (8.2, 9.4)	13.2 (12.2, 14.2)
Sex							
Male	2249	49.6 (46.9,52.2)	4.2 (3.8,4.6)	0.5 (0.3,0.8)	3.4 (3.0,3.9)	8.6 (8.0,9.3)	13.6 (12.5,14.6)
Female	2773	50.4 (47.8,53.1)	4.6 (4.2,5.0)	0.7 (0.4,0.9)	3.8 (3.4,4.2)	9 (8.0,10.0)	12.9 (11.3,14.6)
Indigenous identity							
Non-Indigenous	4937	98.3 (97.4,98.9)	4.4 (4.1,4.7)	0.6 (0.4,0.7)	3.6 (3.3,3.9)	8.8 (8.2,9.4)	13.2 (12.2,14.2)
Indigenous	84	1.7 (1.1,2.6)	3.2 (1.6,4.7)	0.9 * (0.0,1.7)	4.9 (3.2,6.7)	11.5 (7.0,16.0)	14 * (1.9,26.0)
Residential location							
Major cities	2969	72.7 (69.1,76.0)	4 (3.7,4.4)	0.6 (0.4,0.8)	3.4 (3.0,3.8)	8.4 (7.6,9.2)	13.3 (12.0,14.6)
Rural/remote	2053	27.3 (24.0,30.9)	5.4 (4.9,5.9)	0.7 (0.4,1.0)	4.3 (3.7,4.8)	9.6 (8.8,10.3)	13 (11.6,14.4)
Year level of schooling							
Year 10 or less	1190	25.5 (23.5,27.8)	7.7 (7.1,8.2)	0.6 * (0.2,1.0)	4.7 (4.0,5.4)	10.2 (9.4,11.1)	14 (12.5,15.6)
Year 11 or more	3793	74.5 (72.2, 76.5)	3.3 (3.0, 3.5)	0.6 (0.4, 0.7)	3.4 (3.0, 3.8)	7.7 (6.8, 8.6)	11.8 (10.7, 12.9)
Highest qualification attained							
Degree or above	2026	29.3 (26.9,31.8)	2.3 (2.0,2.5)	0.6 (0.3,0.8)	2.4 (2.0,2.7)	6 (5.4,6.6)	11 (9.1,13.0)
Other/None	2931	70.7 (68.2,73.1)	5.3 (4.9,5.6)	0.6 (0.4,0.8)	4.3 (3.9,4.8)	9.4 (8.7,10.1)	13.4 (12.2,14.5)
Eligibility for public dental care							
Eligible	1634	30.7 (28.3,33.1)	7.6 (7.0,8.2)	1 (0.5,1.4)	5.2 (4.5,6.0)	10.1 (9.3,11.0)	13.6 (12.5,14.7)
Ineligible	3373	69.3 (66.9,71.7)	3 (2.7,3.3)	0.5 (0.4,0.6)	3.3 (2.9,3.6)	7.6 (6.7,8.4)	10.8 (9.1,12.5)
Dental insurance							
Insured	2548	45.3 (42.5,48.1)	3.9 (3.5,4.2)	0.4 (0.3,0.6)	3.0 (2.6,3.4)	7.6 (7.0,8.3)	10.8 (9.8,11.8)
Uninsured	2385	54.7 (51.9,57.5)	5 (4.6,5.4)	0.7 (0.5,1.0)	4.3 (3.8,4.8)	9.8 (9.0,10.7)	15 (13.4,16.5)
Usually visit dentist							
For a check-up	3135	61.5 (58.8,64.1)	3.5 (3.2,3.8)	0.5 (0.3,0.7)	3.1 (2.7,3.5)	7.3 (6.8,7.9)	11.3 (10.3,12.3)
For a dental problem	1796	38.5 (35.9,41.2)	6 (5.5,6.5)	0.8 (0.6,1.1)	4.5 (4.0,5.0)	10.6 (9.5,11.7)	16 (14.2,17.8)

* Indicates a relative standard error of at least 25%, and hence should be interpreted with caution.

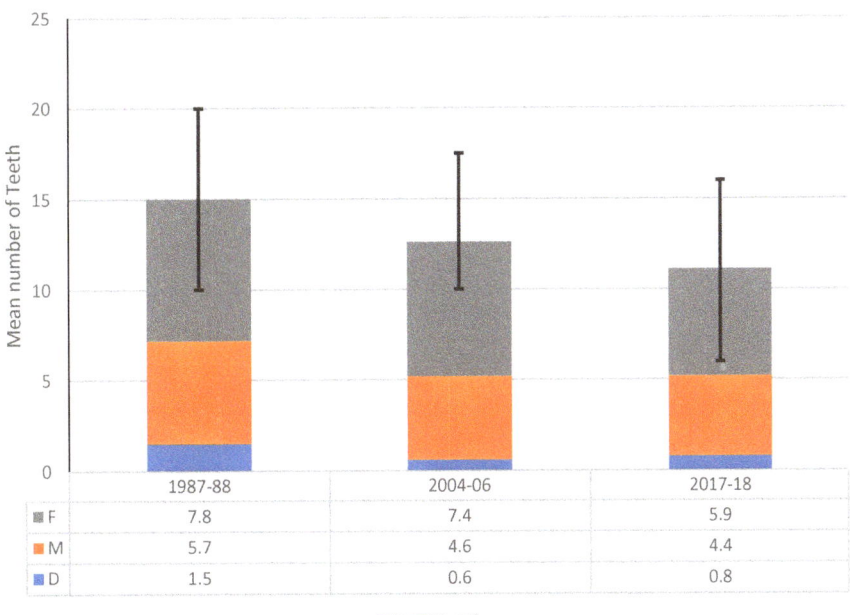

Figure 1. Trends in dental decay experience among dentate Australians aged 15 years and over, 1987–88, 2004–06 and 2017–18.

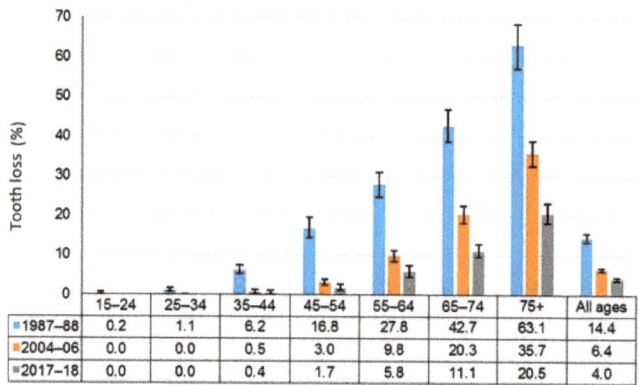

Figure 2. Trends in complete tooth loss among Australians aged 15 years and over, 1987–88, 2004–06 and 2017–18.

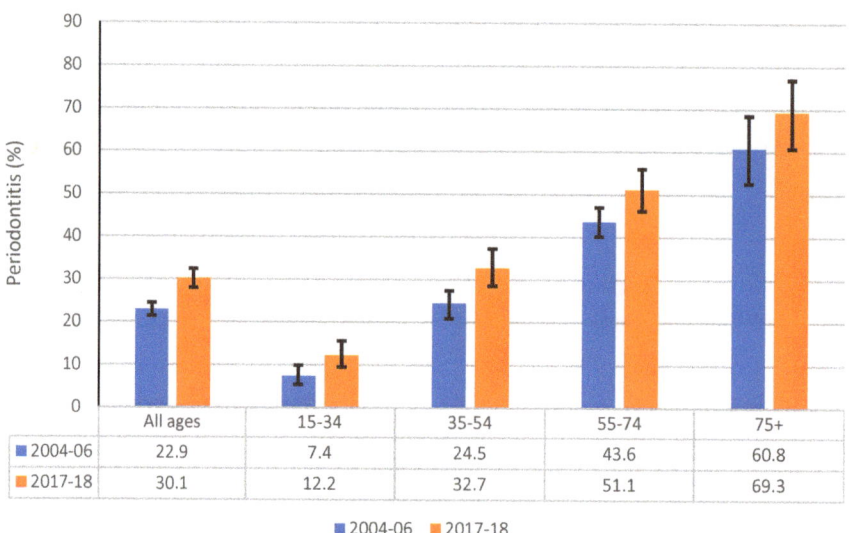

Figure 3. Comparison of the prevalence of moderate or severe periodontitis among dentate Australians aged 15 years and over between 2004–06 and 2017–18.

3.1. Dental Caries

Table 1 shows the proportion of Australian dentate adults aged 15 years and over with untreated coronal caries (one or more decayed surfaces on crowns of their teeth). Nearly one third of Australian adults (32.1%) had at least one tooth surface affected by untreated dental caries. The proportion of adults with dental caries across the four age groups varied, with the prevalence being highest in 35–54-year-olds (35.4%) and lowest among those aged 75 years and over (24.5%). The highest prevalence of untreated dental caries among participants of all ages was reported in those who visited a dentist for a dental problem (43.5%), while participants who visited the dentist for a check-up had the lowest prevalence (24.3%). Higher proportions of untreated dental caries were seen for males, those eligible for public dental care and those without dental insurance. Across age groups, higher proportions were seen for Indigenous people aged 55–74 years and those aged 35–54 years with Year 10 or less level of schooling than their counterparts.

The mean number of decayed tooth surfaces per person in Australian dentate adults aged 15 years and over is presented in Table 2. Overall, Australian dentate adults aged 15 years and over had, on average, 1.4 decayed tooth surfaces. The mean number of decayed tooth surfaces among all ages was lowest in participants who usually visited a dentist for a check-up (0.7), and usually visiting the dentist for a problem was strongly associated with higher mean number of decayed tooth surfaces across all age groups. Those who reported visiting for dental problems had, on average, 2.3 decayed surfaces. In addition, participants who had Year 11 or more schooling, a degree or higher educational qualification, those who were not eligible for public dental care and those with dental insurance had a lower mean number of decayed tooth surfaces than their counterparts.

Table 3 shows the mean number of decayed, missing or filled tooth surfaces (DMFS) per person in the Australian population. On average, Australian dentate adults aged 15 years and over had, on average, 29.7 decayed, missing or filled tooth surfaces, and it increased gradually across four age groups, with people aged ≥75 years having the highest mean DMFS (75.3). Among individuals of all ages, those who were eligible for public dental care had the highest mean DMFS (44.8), and Indigenous people had the lowest mean DMFS (18.7). Moreover, males, individuals with higher levels of schooling and degree or higher qualifications, and those who usually visited a dentist for a check-up had significantly lower mean DMFS as opposed to their counterparts.

3.2. Gingivitis

Table 4 shows the prevalence of gingivitis in the Australian dentate adult population. Overall, 28.8% of Australian dentate adults aged 15 years and over had gingivitis. Although the prevalence of gingivitis was decreasing with age across the four age groups, the differences were not statistically significant. Among all age groups, males had the highest prevalence of gingivitis (34.7%) and females the lowest (23.1%). In addition, those who usually visited a dentist for a dental problem (33.2%) had a greater prevalence of gingivitis than their counterparts.

3.3. Periodontitis

Table 5 presents the percentage of Australian dentate adults aged ≥15 years with moderate/severe periodontitis. Accordingly, the overall prevalence of moderate or severe periodontitis among the Australian dentate population was 30.1%. In contrast to gingivitis, the prevalence of moderate or severe periodontitis significantly increased with age: almost 70% of dentate adults aged ≥75 years experienced periodontitis. The prevalence of periodontitis among participants of all ages was lowest in Indigenous Australians (11.0) and highest in those participants who had Year 10 or less of schooling (45%). Males, individuals without a degree or higher qualification, those who were eligible for public dental care, those not dentally insured and those who usually visited a dentist for a dental problem experienced significantly greater periodontitis levels than their counterparts.

3.4. Tooth Loss

In general, 4% Australian adults aged ≥15 years had lost all their teeth (Table 6). While complete tooth loss was non-existent among the 15–34-year age group, the proportion of adults with complete tooth loss steadily increased from 1.1% among 35–54 year olds to 20.5% for those aged ≥75. Among all age groups, the dentally uninsured had the highest prevalence of complete tooth loss (10.5%), while those who with a degree or above qualification reported the lowest prevalence (0.7%). There was a subtle difference between Indigenous and non-Indigenous adults in regard to complete tooth loss, however, a significantly higher proportion of Indigenous adults aged 55–74 years reported complete tooth loss (29.3%) as opposed to their non-Indigenous equivalents (7.7%). Among all age groups, those with Year 10 or less level of schooling, those without a degree or higher qualification, people who were eligible for public dental care, the dentally uninsured and those who usually visited a dentist for a dental problem had significantly higher levels of complete tooth loss than their counterparts did.

Table 7 shows the severity of tooth loss due to pathology in Australian adults aged 15 years and over. In general, Australian adults had lost, on average, 4.4 teeth due to pathology. The mean number of teeth lost due to pathology increased consistently with age, from 0.6 at 15–34 years to 13.2 at 75 years and above. Among all age groups, the mean number of teeth lost due to pathology was lowest among those who had a degree or above qualification (2.3) and highest among those who were eligible for public dental care (7.7). In addition, people residing in rural/remote areas, those with Year 10 or less level of schooling, those dentally uninsured and those who usually visited a dentist for a dental problem had a significantly higher mean number of teeth lost due to pathology.

3.5. Time Trends in Oral Health

Over the past three decades, three national surveys of adult oral health have been carried out in Australia, namely, the National Oral Health Survey of Australia 1987–88 [18], the National Survey of Adult Oral Health 2004–06 [19], and the National Study of Adult Oral Health 2017–18 [12]. Accordingly, trends in oral health are sourced from these three national surveys, based on three time points. Given comparable data for periodontal disease were not available in the National Oral Health Survey of Australia 1987–88, an analysis of time trends in periodontal disease was not possible. Therefore, only a comparison of the prevalence of moderate or severe periodontitis between 2004–06 and 2017–18 surveys is presented.

Figure 1 presents the trends in the severity of dental caries experience in Australian adults aged $\geq$15, as denoted by mean DMFT. There has been a consistent declining trend in the mean DMFT over 30 years, from 14.9 in 1987–88 to 12.6 and 11.2 in 2004–06 and 2017–18, respectively. It was revealed that substantial reductions in all three components of the mean DMFT over 30 years have contributed to this declining trend. For example, the mean number of decayed teeth (D) and missing teeth due to pathology (M) declined from 1.5 (1987–88) to 0.8 (2017–18) and 5.7 (1987–88) to 4.4 (2017–18), respectively, whereas the average number of filled teeth (F) reduced from 7.8 in 1987–88 to 5.9 in 2017–18.

Figure 2 shows time trends in the proportion of Australian adults with complete tooth loss by age. It is apparent that there has been a steady decline in the overall proportion of Australian adults with complete tooth loss during three time points, from 14.4% in 1987–88 to 6.4% in 2004–06, and to 4% in 2017–18. This decline is reflected across all age groups, particularly among those aged 35–44 years and above, showing substantial reductions in complete tooth loss among them since 1987–88. For instance, there were only 1.7% of individuals aged 45–54 years with complete tooth loss in 2017–18, compared to 16.8% in 1987–88. The proportion of edentulous persons among 55–64-year-olds declined from 27.8% in 1987 to 5.8 in 2017–18. Likewise, nearly one in six adults aged 75+ were edentulous in 1987–88 compared to just one in three in 2017–18.

A comparison of the proportions of Australian adults with moderate or severe periodontitis by age is depicted in Figure 3. The overall prevalence of periodontal disease increased from 22.9% in 2004–06 to 30.1% in 2017–18. This was reflected in a consistent inclination of the proportion of Australian adults affected with periodontal disease across all age groups between 2004–06 and 2017–18. For example, the proportions of Australians aged 15–34 years and 75+ years with periodontitis increased from 7.4% to 12.2% and from 60.8% to 69.3, respectively, between 2004–06 and 2017–18.

4. Discussion

The findings of the present study indicate that overall levels of dental caries and tooth loss among Australian adults have considerably declined over the past three decades. For example, the severity of dental caries experience and complete tooth loss among Australian adults has decreased by nearly 27% and 72%, respectively, from 1987–88 to 2017–18. In general, this decline in dental caries experience has been reflected in all three components of the DMFT index, showing overall reductions of 46%, 22% and 24% in the mean number of decayed, missing and filled teeth over 30 years since 1987–88. In contrast, the periodontal status of Australian adults has substantially deteriorated between 2004–06 and 2017–18, with an overall increase in the prevalence of moderate or severe periodontitis by nearly 31%. This deterioration is evident across all age groups, in particular with the almost 65% increase in the proportion of Australian adults aged 15–34 years who have moderate or severe periodontitis.

Several factors may explain improvements in dental caries experience, as well as tooth retention, that have been observed among Australian adults over the past three decades. Nearly 90% of Australians have access to fluoridated drinking water, while almost 97% of Australian children and adults brushed their teeth daily using a fluoridated toothpaste [20]. There has been consistent evidence to suggest that community water fluoridation alongside widespread use of fluoridated toothpaste in Australia has played the most important role in preventing dental caries [21,22]. Prevention of dental caries in turn has led to increased retention of teeth, given that dental caries is regarded as the main cause of tooth loss. Furthermore, there has been a notable shift in dental treatment strategies, from high-extraction versus low-restoration to low-extraction versus high-restoration, which may have also contributed to improved tooth retention over the past three decades. These findings have consistently shown that Australian adults who usually visited only for a dental problem had higher levels of dental caries and tooth loss than those who visited for a dental check-up. For example, the severity of dental caries (as denoted by the mean DMFT) and the prevalence of complete tooth loss, respectively, were 1.31 and 6.8 times higher among Australian adults who usually visited only for a dental problem than for their counterparts who visited for a dental check-up. This finding concurs with what has been reported previously, indicating an association between improved oral health and favourable dental visiting patterns, including visiting for a dental check-up [23,24].

The NSAOH 2017–18 report has used several independent variables, such as year level of schooling, highest qualification attained, eligibility of public dental care and dental insurance, as socioeconomic indicators of the study population. Accordingly, the present findings have revealed that poor oral health has consistently been associated with lower levels of socioeconomic status. For instance, the prevalence of untreated dental decay was 1.22 times and 1.58 times higher among persons who had Year 10 or less of schooling and those who were dentally uninsured than their counterparts with Year 11 or more years of schooling and those with dental insurance. Likewise, the prevalence of complete tooth loss was 5.26 times and 3.82 times higher among individuals with Year 10 or less schooling and those who were without dental insurance, as opposed to their counterparts. These findings are consistent with those of previous studies, where more socially advantaged individuals presented with much improved oral health levels than those who were worse-off, and, consequently, supported the existence of socioeconomic inequalities in oral health [25,26].

Deterioration in periodontal health in Australian adults, which has been observed between 2004–06 and 2017–18, could be mainly ascribed to increased tooth retention. While the overall proportion of edentulous persons declined from 6.4% to 4%, the mean number of missing teeth due to pathology dropped from 4.6 to 4.4 during this period. Consequently, both the increase in the proportion of dentate adults as well as the number of retained teeth pose a greater vulnerability for periodontal disease. Our findings were consistent with those of previous studies where a strong association between age and periodontitis was observed; the older the individuals, the higher the prevalence of periodontal disease [10]. Associations between socioeconomic variables and periodontal disease, on the other hand, were similar to those seen with regard to dental caries and tooth loss. Accordingly, the prevalence of moderate or severe periodontitis was consistently higher among Australian adults in the lower socioeconomic strata. This is consistent with previous studies [10] and provides further evidence for the presence of socioeconomic disparities in oral health.

Employing a nationally representative sample of Australian adults and using a standardized examination protocol, as well as rigorous epidemiological survey methods, were some of the main strengths of the study. Other strengths included having both the interviewers and oral examiners adequately trained to ensure the quality control of the study (high intra-class correlation coefficient values were obtained indicating a high level of inter-examiner reliability and agreement), and the instruments used were based on previous studies, enabling comparisons to be made across the series of national surveys. Whilst the cross-sectional nature of the study did not warrant ascertaining cause–effect relationships, the present study could not represent Indigenous Australians in sufficient numbers. This, in turn, has resulted in creating small cell counts and relative standard errors of at least 25% in regard to Indigenous group/subgroup analyses, so interpretation of these results should be made with caution. Moreover, the use of partial recording protocols in the study could have contributed to flaws in estimating the prevalence of periodontitis. Despite such limitations, the findings showed that the overall oral health status, including the experience of dental caries, periodontal disease and tooth loss, was poorer in Indigenous Australians than in their non-Indigenous counterparts with regard to virtually all independent variables assessed. These findings are consistent with the previous studies, which were conducted among Indigenous groups in both Australia and elsewhere, indicating that Indigenous populations are among the most socioeconomically disadvantaged communities in the world [27–29]. It may be challenging for survey instruments and sampling methods employed in conventional population-level oral health surveys to capture the true picture of Indigenous populations and, accordingly, the need for implementing unique study methodologies for such populations has been highlighted [29].

5. Conclusions

The present findings suggest that the overall oral health, barring periodontal status, of Australian adults has improved over the last 30 years. Comparisons of national data between 2004–06 and 2017–18 reveal that the periodontal health of Australian adults, in general, has deteriorated during this period. The findings also indicate that individuals from lower socioeconomic backgrounds present with poorer oral health on the whole, pointing to socioeconomic inequalities in oral health. Such findings may be useful for policy makers in planning and implementing future oral healthcare programmes at a population level.

Author Contributions: Conceptualization, N.A., L.L., S.C. and L.M.J.; formal analysis, S.C. and N.A.; writing—original draft preparation, N.A.; writing—review and editing, N.A., L.L., S.C. and L.M.J. All authors have read and agreed to the published version of the manuscript.

Funding: This research was funded by the Australian Government Department of Health and the National Health and Medical Research Council (Partnership Grant #1115649).

Institutional Review Board Statement: This study was reviewed and approved by The University of Adelaide's Human Research Ethics Committee (HREC; H-2016-046).

Informed Consent Statement: Interviewed subjects provided verbal consent prior to answering questions. Parental/guardian consent was obtained for participants aged 15–17 years. All examined subjects provided signed, informed consent prior to the examination (parents/guardians of those aged 15–17 years provided signed, informed consent prior to the examination).

Data Availability Statement: The datasets used during the current study are available from the corresponding author via completion of a data request.

Acknowledgments: The Australian Dental Association, Colgate Oral Care and BUPA provided sponsorship. State/Territory health departments and dental services were partners in the study. The research team acknowledge the Australian Government Department of Human Services, state and territory dental health services and the participants involved in the study.

Conflicts of Interest: The authors declare no conflict of interest.

References

1. World Health Organization. Regional Office for Europe. 2021. Available online: https://www.euro.who.int/en/health-topics/disease-prevention/oral-health (accessed on 4 July 2021).
2. Glick, M.; Williams, D.M.; Kleinman, D.V.; Vujicic, M.; Watt, R.G.; Weyant, R.J. A new definition for oral health developed by the FDI World Dental Federation opens the door to a universal definition of oral health. *J. Public Health Dent.* **2017**, *77*, 3–5. [CrossRef] [PubMed]
3. Lee, J.Y.; Watt, R.G.; Williams, D.M.; Giannobile, W.V. A New Definition for Oral Health: Implications for Clinical Practice, Policy, and Research. *J. Dent. Res.* **2017**, *96*, 125–127. [CrossRef] [PubMed]
4. Seymour, B.; James, Z.; Shroff Karhade, D.; Barrow, J.; Pruneddu, A.; Anderson, N.K.; Mossey, P. Definition of Global Health TFFT. A definition of global oral health: An expert consensus approach by the Consortium of Universities for Global Health's Global Oral Health Interest Group. *Glob. Health Action* **2020**, *13*, 1814001. [CrossRef] [PubMed]
5. World Health Organization. Oral Health. 2021. Available online: https://www.who.int/news-room/fact-sheets/detail/oral-health (accessed on 6 July 2021).
6. Peres, M.A.; Macpherson, L.M.D.; Weyant, R.J.; Daly, B.; Venturelli, R.; Mathur, M.; Listl, S.; Celeste, R.K.; Guarnizo-Herreño, C.C.; Kearns, C.; et al. Oral diseases: A global public health challenge. *Lancet* **2019**, *394*, 249–260. [CrossRef]
7. Veiga, N.; Aires, D.; Douglas, F.; Pereira, M.; Vaz, A.; Rama, L.; Silva, P.; Miranda, V.; Pereira, F.; Vidal, B.; et al. Dental caries: A review. *J. Dent. Oral Health* **2016**, *2*, 1–3.
8. GBD 2016 Causes of Death Collaborators. Global, regional, and national age-sex specific mortality for 264 causes of death, 1980–2016, a systematic analysis for the Global Burden of Disease Study 2016. *Lancet* **2017**, *390*, 1151–1210. [CrossRef]
9. GBD 2017 Causes of Death Collaborators. Global, regional, and national age-sex-specific mortality for 282 causes of death in 195 countries and territories, 1980–2017, a systematic analysis for the Global Burden of Disease Study 2017. *Lancet* **2018**, *392*, 1736–1788. [CrossRef]
10. Kassebaum, N.J.; Bernabé, E.; Dahiya, M.; Bhandari, B.; Murray, C.J.; Marcenes, W. Global burden of severe periodontitis in 1990–2010, a systematic review and meta-regression. *J. Dent. Res.* **2014**, *93*, 1045–1053. [CrossRef] [PubMed]
11. Australian Institute of Health and Welfare. Oral Health and Dental Care in Australia. Cat. no. DEN 231; AIHW: Canberra, Australia, 2021. Available online: https://www.aihw.gov.au/reports/dental-oral-health/oral-health-and-dental-care-in-australia/contents/healthy-teeth (accessed on 27 July 2021).
12. Australian Research Centre for Population Oral Health (ARCPOH). *Australia's Oral Health: The National Study of Adult Oral Health 2017–18*; University of Adelaide: Adelaide, Australia, 2019.
13. Chrisopoulos, S.; Ellershaw, E.; Luzzi, L. National Study of Adult Oral Health 2017–2018, Study design and methods. *Aust. Dent. J.* **2020**, *65*, S5–S10. [CrossRef] [PubMed]
14. Stewart, J.F.; Ellershaw, A. *Oral Health and Use of Dental Services 2008. Findings from the National Dental Telephone Interview Survey 2008*; Dental Statistics and Research Series no. 58. Cat. no. DEN 216; Australian Institute if Health and Welfare: Canberra, Australia, 2012.
15. Do, L.G.; Peres, K.G.; Ha, D.H.; Roberts-Thomson, K. Oral epidemiological examination—Protocol: The National Study of Adult Oral Health 2017–18. *Aust. Dent. J.* **2020**, *65*, S18–S22. [CrossRef] [PubMed]
16. Loe, H.; Silness, J. Periodontal disease in pregnancy. I. Prevalence and severity. *Acta Odontol. Scand.* **1963**, *21*, 533–551. [CrossRef] [PubMed]
17. NIDCR. *National Health and Nutrition Examination Survey Dental Examiners Procedures Manual*; US National Center for Health Statistics: Hyattsville, MD, USA, 2002.
18. Barnard, P.D. *National Oral Health Survey Australia 1987–88*; Australian Government Publishing Services: Canberra, Australia, 1993.
19. Roberts-Thomson, K.; Do, L. *Australia's Dental Generations: The National Survey of Adult Oral Health 2004–2006*; Australian Institute of Health and Welfare: Canberra, Australia, 2007.
20. Australian Institute of Health and Welfare. *Australia's National Oral Health Plan 2015–2024, Performance Monitoring Report in Brief*; Cat. no. DEN 234; AIHW: Canberra, Australia, 2020.
21. Do, L.G. Australian Research Centre for Population Oral Health. Guidelines for use of fluorides in Australia: Update 2019. *Aust. Dent. J.* **2020**, *65*, 30–38. [CrossRef] [PubMed]
22. Spencer, A.J.; Liu, P.; Armfield, J.M.; Do, L.G. Preventive benefit of access to fluoridated water for young adults. *J. Public Health Dent.* **2017**, *77*, 263–271. [CrossRef] [PubMed]
23. Thomson, W.M.; Williams, S.M.; Broadbent, J.M.; Poulton, R.; Locker, D. Long-term dental visiting patterns and adult oral health. *J. Dent. Res.* **2010**, *89*, 307–311. [CrossRef] [PubMed]
24. Amarasena, N.; Kapellas, K.; Skilton, M.R.; Maple-Brown, L.J.; Brown, A.; Bartold, M.; O'Dea, K.; Celermajer, D.; Jamieson, L.M. Factors Associated with Routine Dental Attendance among Aboriginal Australians. *J. Health Care Poor Underserved* **2016**, *27* (Suppl. 1), 67–80. [CrossRef] [PubMed]
25. Sanders, A.E. *Social Determinants of Oral Health: Conditions Linked to Socioeconomic Inequalities in Oral Health and in the Australian Population*; Population Oral Health Series No. 7; Australian Institute of Health and Welfare: Canberra, Australia, 2007.
26. Mejia, G.C.; Elani, H.W.; Harper, S.; Thomson, W.M.; Ju, X.; Kawachi, I.; Kaufman, J.S.; Jamieson, L.M. Socioeconomic status, oral health and dental disease in Australia, Canada, New Zealand and the United States. *BMC Oral Health* **2018**, *18*, 176. [CrossRef] [PubMed]

27. Amarasena, N.; Kapellas, K.; Skilton, M.R.; Maple-Brown, L.J.; Brown, A.; O'Dea, K.; Celermajer, D.; Jamieson, L.M. Associations with dental caries experience among a convenience sample of Aboriginal Australian adults. *Aust. Dent. J.* **2015**, *60*, 471–478. [CrossRef] [PubMed]
28. Jamieson, L.M.; Elani, H.W.; Mejia, G.C.; Ju, X.; Kawachi, I.; Harper, S.; Thomson, W.M.; Kaufman, J.S. Inequalities in Indigenous Oral Health: Findings from Australia, New Zealand, and Canada. *J. Dent. Res.* **2016**, *95*, 1375–1380. [CrossRef] [PubMed]
29. Jamieson, L.; Hedges, J.; Peres, M.A.; Guarnizo-Herreño, C.C.; Bastos, J.L. Challenges in identifying indigenous peoples in population oral health surveys: A commentary. *BMC Oral Health* **2021**, *21*, 216. [CrossRef]

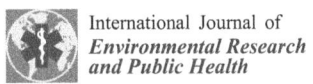

Review

Fit for Purpose—Re-Designing Australia's Mental Health Information System

Sebastian Rosenberg [1],*, Luis Salvador-Carulla [2], Graham Meadows [3] and Ian Hickie [1]

1. Brain and Mind Centre, University of Sydney, Level 4, 94 Mallett Street, Sydney, NSW 2050, Australia; ian.hickie@sydney.edu.au
2. Mental Health Policy Unit, Health Research Institute, Faculty of Health, University of Canberra, Canberra, ACT 2617, Australia; luis.salvador-carulla@canberra.edu.au
3. Department of Psychiatry, Monash Health, Melbourne, VIC 3168, Australia; graham.meadows@monash.edu
* Correspondence: sebastian.rosenberg@sydney.edu.au

Citation: Rosenberg, S.; Salvador-Carulla, L.; Meadows, G.; Hickie, I. Fit for Purpose—Re-Designing Australia's Mental Health Information System. *Int. J. Environ. Res. Public Health* **2022**, *19*, 4808. https://doi.org/10.3390/ijerph19084808

Academic Editor: Richard Madden

Received: 25 January 2022
Accepted: 11 April 2022
Published: 15 April 2022

Publisher's Note: MDPI stays neutral with regard to jurisdictional claims in published maps and institutional affiliations.

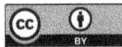

Copyright: © 2022 by the authors. Licensee MDPI, Basel, Switzerland. This article is an open access article distributed under the terms and conditions of the Creative Commons Attribution (CC BY) license (https://creativecommons.org/licenses/by/4.0/).

Abstract: Background: Monitoring and reporting mental health is complex. Australia's first National Mental Health Strategy in 1992 included a new national commitment to accountability and data collection in mental health. This article provides a narrative review of thirty years of experience. Materials and Methods: This review considers key documents, policies, plans and strategies in relation to the evolution of mental health data and reporting. Documents produced by the Federal and the eight state and territory governments are considered, as well as publications produced by key information agencies, statutory authorities and others. A review of this literature demonstrates both its abundance and limitations. Results: Australia's approach to mental health reporting is characterised by duplication and a lack of clarity. The data available fail to do justice to the mental health services provided in Australia. Mental health data collection and reporting processes are centrally driven, top–down and activity-focused, largely eschewing actual health outcomes, the social determinants of mental health. There is little, if any, link to clearly identifiable service user or carer priorities. Consequently, it is difficult to link this process longitudinally to clinical or systemic quality improvement. Initial links between the focus of national reform efforts and mental health data collection were evident, but these links have weakened over time. Changes to governance and reporting, including under COVID, have made the task of delivering accountability for mental health more difficult. Conclusion: Australia's current approach is not fit for purpose. It is at a pivotal point in mental health reform, with new capacity to use modelled data to simulate prospective mental health reform options. By drawing on these new techniques and learning the lessons of the past, Australia (and other nations) can design and implement more effective systems of planning, reporting and accountability for mental health.

Keywords: mental health; accountability; quality improvement; policy development

1. Introduction

What does effective national monitoring and reporting of mental health care look like? The year 2022 is the thirtieth anniversary of Australia's National Mental Health Strategy, which implemented a new process for data collection as a central function to drive better accountability for mental health services [1].

This narrative review attempts to assess the extent to which Australia's efforts have yielded an effective system of accountability for mental health. This assessment is problematic. There has never been any formal evaluation of the strategy overall. Initial markers of success were not described to permit simple evaluation of progress. Evidence of impact, if available at all, is typically qualitative or summative, not quantitative.

There are some strengths, but also many weaknesses, in the approach taken. This has delivered an Australian reporting system which predominantly focuses on administrative data, inputs and outputs. Much is known about budgets, the number of occupied beds and outpatient occasions of services. We know staffing numbers and costs. However, few details are known about who is presenting for mental health care and why. We also know little about the type of interventions provided or their outcomes and the subsequent pathway taken by patients. Our view of key issues outside of the health sector, in areas such as housing, education and employment, is very limited. We are not able to compare or benchmark services, meaning that our system of accountability fails to impel systemic quality improvement.

As if accountability for mental health was not complex enough, past decades have seen mental health subject to multiple reforms and overlapping reporting processes. This paper traces this history and its impact on Australia's efforts to establish effective accountability across two national mental health policies, five national mental health plans, one national action plan, several other national documents, one roadmap and multiple statutory inquiries over the past three decades. More recently, COVID-19 has seen Australia's Federal government establish a new National Cabinet, scrapping previous administrative structures which oversaw accountability for mental health, such as the Australian Health Ministers Council [2].

Federal, state and territory governments are currently arranging bilateral agreements which will constitute the backbone of Australia's sixth national mental health plan, including specifying data and reporting obligations. It would be folly to assume the utility of existing reporting arrangements. Indeed, under the maxim 'what gets measured gets done', there is reason to be alert to the risk of poor data collection processes reinforcing undesirable models of care. For example, if hospital beds are the currency reported, beds will remain the priority for policy and funding, regardless of the merits of alternatives.

Understanding Australia's historical approach to mental health reporting can inform the next steps and help drive the development of more robust processes designed to deliver national accountability.

2. Materials and Methods

While no formal evaluation of Australia's National Mental Health Strategy has occurred, this does not mean that there is a paucity of evidence. Comments and critiques are plentiful, generated by the frequent statutory, parliamentary and other inquiries commonplace over the past two decades. One report suggested that there had been thirty-two separate statutory or other inquiries between 2006 and 2012 alone [3]. Such inquiries relying on qualitative or summative evidence have often been initiated in response to deaths, human rights abuses or other tragedies. While they do not purport to formally evaluate the National Mental Health Strategy as a whole, they frequently touch on accountability and monitoring, making them worthy of consideration and review here.

In this context, this paper has relied on a narrative review, aiming to present a comprehensive, critical analysis of current knowledge in relation to Australia's approach to reporting and accountability for mental health. It is possible, on this basis, to discern gaps and patterns, as well as strengths and weaknesses, in the data [4].

Key documents, policies, plans and strategies are considered, demonstrating the evolution of mental health data and reporting. Historical documents are cited, including several which highlight implications arising from our federated system of government. Government and statutory reports, as well as peer-reviewed and other literature (from grey literature, websites, media sources, etc.) are referenced. The jumble of reports and inquiries needs a timeline to orient readers, and this is presented. The paper explores recent recommendations made by various reports and how these can influence the direction of future reforms. It then draws on contemporary literature to describe the components of an effective, contemporary approach to accountability for mental health.

What Is Meant by Accountability?

Accountability is an elusive concept, with multiple valid perspectives [5]. Planners would like to know the value for money. Service providers wish to understand if their work has been effective and how it could be improved. Consumers and families want to know what services and treatments work. Funders want information about cost-effectiveness and value for money, using systems such as activity-based funding to generate costs and prices and monitor system efficiency [6,7]. Researchers will want data to evaluate or compare alternative approaches, programs or services.

The community more generally will want information indicating the extent to which it has access to a mental health system that responds to individual needs and is one on which it can rely.

In relation to health care generally, accountability can increase the effectiveness of services, reduce inefficiency and provide the feedback necessary to impel systemic quality improvement [8,9].

The data generated for accountability are commonly considered across three dimensions: financial, performance and political/democratic [10]. Financial accountability relates to ensuring that funds are spent as agreed, monitoring, auditing and budgeting.

Performance accountability can refer to the assessment of services, outputs or outcomes, allowing value for money to be assessed. Political accountability is often focused on whether governments kept their promises, often with reference to notions of equity, efficiency and so on.

These perspectives on accountability overlap, but stakeholders may prioritise data differently. This diversity again lends itself to the narrative method of analysis used throughout this discussion.

3. Results

3.1. Initial Efforts in Mental Health Information

The 1992 National Mental Health Strategy, which included an overarching policy and a plan, had data and accountability at its heart (Box 1).

Box 1. Extract from 1992 National Mental Health Policy.

> There needs to be greater accountability and visibility in reporting progress in implementing the new national approach to mental health services. Currently mental health data collection is inconsistent and would not be adequate to enable an assessment to be made of the relative stage of development of the Commonwealth and each State/Territory Government in achieving the objectives outlined in the National mental health policy. It is essential that such a consistent system of monitoring and accountability be created.
>
> *National Mental Health Policy (Commonwealth of Australia 1992)*

The aim of this novel approach to accountability for mental health was to report on the progress being made by governments against the Strategy's agreed goals.

The Australian Health Ministers' Council established a working group to oversee the implementation of the Strategy. The National Mental Health Working Group was comprised of representatives from each state and territory, plus two from the Federal government, as well as the chair and deputy chair of the newly established National Community Advisory Group, which included consumers and carers. This working group established a set of 49 indicators to fulfil the accountability monitoring function recommended in the policy.

However, the data required to report against many of these indicators either did not exist or were not collected. The working group established a Mental Health Information Strategy Sub-Committee (MHISSC) [11] comprised of the same representation as the working group plus representatives from the Australian Bureau of Statistics (ABS), the Australian Institute of Health and Welfare (AIHW) and the Australian Private Hospitals' Association. The MHISSC developed a National Mental Health Data Dictionary and Minimum Data Set for Australia.

The MHISSC oversaw the development of a specific new data collection process designed to fulfil the Working Group's mental health reporting obligations under the Policy. This was conducted outside the structures established already by the National Health Information Agreement, which provided the framework for establishing national data collections and data standards [12].

The Federal government engaged consultants to manage the process of collecting and analysing data, and then published a series of National Mental Health Reports [13] to draw together material from all jurisdictions, as well as the private sector.

After a baseline was established in 1993, the first report was published in 1994 [14]. By the time the Commonwealth decided to cease the series, twelve editions had been produced. The final National Mental Health Report (2013) used 18 graphs or tables to describe the pace of reform [13].

This report, produced separately from other existing health data and by external consultants, became the key tool by which the community could track changes in the shape and nature of mental health care. Drawing on the definition provided earlier, the National Mental Health Report series had a clear focus on political accountability, purporting to enable governments to answer the question "Did we do what we agreed?" [13].

Over time, the collection and report became more robust, with data elements incorporated into different national minimum datasets [15]. It reflected a strong focus on the role of the states and territories as the main providers of care, for example, in delivering the policy goal of 'mainstreaming' mental health services.

The reporting also had a heavy emphasis on financial accountability, as described earlier, reporting inputs such as spending and staffing, and outputs, as well as administrative data, such as treatment days, the number of services and clients.

The collection was not designed to drive a process of systemic quality improvement, nor reflect perspectives on accountability held by mental health stakeholders, such as consumers or even health professionals. Stakeholders from across the mental health sector and outside of the government would prioritise accountability issues and questions different to those selected by the government [16].

3.2. Limited Aims, Limited Performance

The pursuit of even this rather limited dataset was challenging enough—obtaining agreement on data collection standards and definitions between nine Australian jurisdictions is difficult. The process requires consensus across governments [17].

MHISSC then had to oversee the process by which each government obtained, vetted and cleaned the necessary data. This governmental approval was a slow process, causing delays in publication. For example, the data published in the 2013 National Mental Health Report pertained to the 2010–2011 financial year. This lag has not improved. In 2022, the AIHW's Mental Health Services in Australia website [18], now the key data resource, is still only able to report mental health expenditure up until 2018–2019.

There was no independent verification of the data provided to the Report and, particularly in the first years, the quality and range of data varied between jurisdictions. There was no way to marry annual mental health budget allocations to the actual expenditure or to the costs of services. These matters limited the extent to which data could be usefully interpreted for benchmarking between jurisdictions.

The data were only published at the jurisdictional level (i.e., by state and territory). This could be useful, revealing how the shape and nature of the mental health services available differ between the states. For example, the 2013 National Report showed that Tasmania offered 19.5 beds per 100,000 inhabitants in residential mental health care settings, while Queensland provided zero. However, the Report had no capacity to provide data at more disaggregated levels, preventing a more detailed and regional comparison of service patterns or other issues [13].

The 1997 Evaluation of the first national mental health plan, while noting the role of the National Mental Health Report, stated:

> *Information in mental health is grossly undeveloped. The lack of nationally comparable data on service outputs, costs, quality and outcomes places major limitations on the extent to which the National Mental Health Strategy can achieve its objectives.* [19]

An initial $135 m investment made by the then Federal Government to sponsor reform and accountability under the First Plan was not replicated in subsequent plans [20].

Key proponents of the national reforms noted that, under the Second National Mental Health Plan, momentum "waned" [21].

A decade later, the 'summative' evaluation of the 3rd National Mental Health Plan (2003–2008) repeated concerns about national monitoring and reporting mechanisms, suggesting that there was duplication, waste and an inability to measure appropriate outcome measures [22].

These concerns about data and accountability processes in mental health were echoed in repeated statutory reports and inquiries [23,24]. A report jointly prepared by the Human Rights and Equal Opportunity Commission and the [then] Mental Health Council of Australia found:

> *The National Mental Health Strategy was developed over a decade ago to respond to obvious service failures and human rights concerns....we do not yet have a national process for translating the policy rhetoric into real increases in resources, enhanced service access, accepted service standards or service accountability.* [25]

3.3. Fragmentation of Effort, Minimal Improvement

The ownership of responsibility for national mental health reporting shifted in 2006 from health ministers to first ministers, with the Council of Australian Governments (CoAG) agreeing to a $5.5 bn National Action Plan on Mental Health [26]. The rationale for the CoAG's involvement is not entirely clear. There were two damning inquiries which required some political response [23,25]. The CoAG itself reported that its engagement was based on "a broad recognition that renewed government effort was needed to give greater impetus to the reform process" [26]. The Action Plan brought together the heads of all governments to focus on mental health for the first time and included its own list of outcomes and progress measures.

The CoAG's list had greater emphasis on social indicators, such as employment and education, than the mental health service indicators prioritised by the MHISSC. It also reflected greater engagement by the Federal government in mental health service provision. The CoAG Action Plan generated progress reports, again designed for the government to fulfil a level of political accountability and demonstrate "Are we doing what we said we would?" [27].

There were several other reports and inquiries into mental health emerging in quick succession that recommended changes to the way data are reported, or even proposed new sets of indicators [24,28] (see Table A1 for a timeline). These recommendations were not actioned.

The process of providing national accountability oversight in mental health has become increasingly confused with multiple overlapping initiatives, policies, plans and datasets. This has dramatically increased the gap between planning and reporting, and actual action and monitoring of mental health. Key processes identified as part of effective policy development and evaluation are missing [29].

The 2012 National Mental Health Roadmap, for example, listed 11 'performance' indicators and 3 'contextual' indicators [30]. The 4th National Mental Health Plan and associated Implementation and Measurement Strategies listed 25 indicators [31]. It continued the CoAG's emphasis on broader measures of the social determinants of mental health, promising a "whole of government approach" so that:

> *The public is able to make informed judgements about the extent of mental health reform in Australia, including the progress of the fourth plan, and has confidence in the information available to make these judgements. Consumers and carers have access to*

information about the performance of services responsible for their care across the range of health quality domains and are able to compare these to national benchmarks [32].

The National Mental Health Commission began in 2012 and soon produced its own annual National Mental Health Report [33] drawing on frameworks, indicators, case studies and stories, rather than against a consistent dataset. In 2014, the Commission was tasked with a review of mental health programs and services and reported, in 2015, on a lack of outcome-based evaluation data and accountability mechanisms [34]. It recommended a focus on a much smaller number of indicators, focusing much more on outcomes than outputs, together with a transition to a much more regionally based system of planning and reporting. The Commission's recommendations remain unimplemented.

The impetus towards greater accountability in mental health in relation to its social determinants was affirmed in the 2014 strategic plan of the NSW Mental Health Commission, which reported that spending on mental health by the NSW Department of Family and Community Services was greater than that by the NSW Department of Health [35]. Accountability for health care alone cannot provide a true picture of mental health.

Despite this, the 5th National Mental Health and Suicide Prevention Plan [36] and its accompanying Implementation Plan (2017) [37] promised monitoring and reporting around a more limited set of 24 core health indicators, focusing on safety and quality.

This Plan promised to draw on proxy data to deal with social determinant issues as part of this, for example, using the Australian Bureau of Statistics General Social Survey to report the social participation of people with a mental illness.

Leaving aside issues such as resources or political will, the infrastructure to support good data collection in mental health has been slow to evolve. Several other countries have developed sophisticated maps [38], permitting benchmarking and the comparison of key mental health services between jurisdictions. Such maps are new to Australia and are not yet driving decision-making. Alternative classifications and structures, such as the Australian Classification of Health Interventions (ACHI), have been demonstrated to be less than comprehensive when applied to mental health [39].

The history of Australian efforts in relation to data collection and reporting has left us with at best a partial picture—strong in relation to health and administrative data, but weak in other areas, particularly outside of hospitals and in relation to the broader social determinants of mental health. It is a situation described as "outcome blind" [40].

3.4. Other Key Reporting Mechanisms in Mental Health

There are two other key sources of mental health data in Australia. Unlike the National Strategy reporting, both have demonstrated some consistency.

The Australian Institute of Health and Welfare (AIHW) has published the Mental Health Services in Australia (MHSIA) data series since 1988–1999 [18], drawing on the National Mental Health Data Dictionary and Minimum Data Set originally developed by the MHISSC.

Other national minimum data sets have been developed and become part of MHSIA reporting, including in relation to:

- Mental health establishments;
- Admitted patient care;
- Residential mental health care;
- Community mental health care;
- Causes of death (for suicide data).

In 2021, this array of data permits the publication of 35 tables of information. The AIHW also hold and manage an 'indicator library' [41] from which they derived a set of 26 Key Performance Indicators, including issues such as rates of seclusion and restraint, rates of access to mental health care, community contact pre- and post-discharge, etc. [42]. The AIHW was also the manager of the National Mental Health Performance Framework [43] until the cessation of the CoAG in 2020.

The Productivity Commission prepares the Report on Government Services which, for 25 years, has included a section on mental health services [44,45]. Around 60 tables of information are published each year online, providing data at the state and territory levels across 13 key indicators.

There is considerable overlap across the AIHW and Productivity Commission reporting—they both provide data on public mental health service data, expenditure, staffing and access. Additionally, both publications focus on the health service aspect of mental health care, rather than the broader social determinants. They use proxy data derived from general community survey information to estimate and report on matters such as housing and employment. Both suffer from considerable delays in publication. They report progress at the jurisdictional level, permitting, for example, a comparison of the proportion of all mental health-related emergency department presentations in public hospitals between Western Australia and Tasmania. The work of the AIHW and the Productivity Commission in reporting mental health data, even at this level, is helpful, but, as recommended by the Productivity Commission Review (see below), more useful comparisons need to be established between regions, not between states [46]. This more granular approach reflects the fact that regions may have more in common and provide more valid benchmarks than comparing whole jurisdictions, such as Victoria and NSW.

3.5. The Productivity Commission Review 2020

The report found duplication and a lack of clarity in mental health reporting arrangements and called for all governments to agree on a new set of realistic measures and outcomes. It suggested a new framework with six key areas and 47 identified indicators [46]. This was echoed by the Victorian Royal Commission, which reported in 2021 that:

System leadership is weak, and accountability for how the system is managed is unclear. [47]

These findings are obviously a strong indictment of the approach taken in Australia so far.

Under various reporting structures, the MHISSC operated continuously until the Council of Australian Governments (CoAG) was disbanded in May 2020 in favour of new National Cabinet reporting arrangements. Thus far, these arrangements seem rudimentary.

Eleven general health issues are listed under a 'Performance Reporting Dashboard', of which one pertains to mental health. However, rather than provide any data or indicators, what is presented is simply a list of some projects undertaken in each jurisdiction under a green tick symbol and the word "Achieved" [48].

The final National Mental Health Report was published in 2013. There have been no evaluations of either the 4th or 5th National Mental Health Plans and, as stated, no evaluation of the Strategy overall. Despite the regular calls for annual and transparent reporting and monitoring of progress, there is no current system or process for this to occur.

In 2021, the Federal Government released its response to the Productivity Commission report [49], undertaking with the states and territories to establish a new National Agreement on Mental Health and Suicide Prevention by November 2021.

4. Discussion

Lessons Learned—Towards a Better Process of Accountability and Planning

From the experiences of the past thirty years, several important trends and challenges have emerged in relation to how Australia and other nations can engineer more effective and useful data collection and accountability for mental health. In recognition of the increasing role and potential of primary and community-based mental health care, new datasets continue to emerge, requiring intelligent amalgamation with existing systems to exploit new opportunities [50,51]. There is merit in considering how these issues might shape a new process or framework for mental health reporting and planning.

Improved reporting must finally accept the significance of understanding not just basic inputs and outputs, but the whole mental health 'ecosystem' [52], drawing on a broader set of metrics which properly reflect the mental health and wellbeing of communities. This poses new problems in organising and gathering requisite data from multiple agencies, not just health departments. The coordination of this kind of whole-of-government monitoring was one rationale for several jurisdictions to establish mental health commissions [53].

As stated, the issue of regional data is increasingly recognised as key to enabling better local planning in mental health. Despite commitments made to establish regular benchmarking in mental health over past decades [20,54], the establishment and reporting of data at this level is not yet a feature of mental health reporting in Australia, though the AIHW publication of Medicare data by statistical local area (SLA) is an exception [55]. Australia's failure to develop a suitable mental health performance management framework with agreed, consistent indicators and targets has been pinpointed as a key drawback to reform [46].

Engaging mental health stakeholders in developing such a framework would build an understanding of the process and confidence in the results [56]. To date, MHISSC and associated governments have been largely responsible for determining how mental health is reported. MHISSC relied for twenty years on external consultants to manage the process of data collection and reporting [57]. The benefits of broadening this process have been recognised [46]. Specific mention must be made of consumers and carers in this context. The National Community Advisory Group (NCAG) mentioned earlier was disbanded after just three years in 1996. Structures to engage consumers and carers in framework co-design will require considerable development [58].

Another design element should be the widespread use of new personal technologies which permit services users to be the key reporters of real-time and local data pertaining to their care [59], as has already been demonstrated both in Australia [60] and elsewhere [61]. This should be part of a fundamental re-design of accountability for mental health, one that recognises the broader social context of mental illness beyond health, considering issues such as employment, education completion and social connectedness. Despite some initiatives [62], Australia still lacks a validated, national collection of the experience of care of mental health consumers and carers.

Finally, the way mental health is reported relates to how it is planned, and this is a matter currently up for national debate. Historic, centralised approaches to planning are being challenged by more local or regional models of governance and decision-making, as encouraged by the Productivity Commission [46] and the National Mental Health Commission.

There are new decision-support systems which enable this local planning and modelling [63–65]. There are clearly limitations in the extent to which existing state and territory-focused mental health data collections can provide the information these new models need to facilitate better local decision-making, or what other information might be necessary. The examination and resolution of these issues is a key element of more effective planning and reporting of mental health care.

Key bodies internationally have recognised the inability of existing mental health data systems to propel the desired processes of benchmarking and quality improvement [66]. They have embarked on projects designed to make mental health data systems more robust and useful. The World Health Organisation has, for example, prioritised the creation of a mental health data platform aiming at routinely collected information on mental health systems' performance and on the mental health status of the population. These Australian lessons could inform this work [67].

The Australian experience demonstrates the importance of establishing an accurate historical account of the evolution of the core policy and planning processes underpinning mental health reform, giving context and meaning to the status of national and regional mental health systems. Our experience has shown how complicated this process can be, even in countries with significant resources.

5. Conclusions

Australia has not produced a comprehensive report or evaluation of its national mental health planning effort. This means that, despite myriad plans and reports, it is not possible to assess the extent to which this work has translated into effective change, the costs, nor the impact on individual outcomes or systemic improvement.

Even where partial data have been reported, there was no independent verification of the data provided and, particularly in the first years, the quality and range of data varied between jurisdictions. There was no way to marry annual mental health budget allocations to actual expenditure or to the costs of services. These matters limited the extent to which data could be usefully interpreted for benchmarking between jurisdictions. Australia has lacked consistent data sets. Overlapping reports, indicator sets and report cards have perpetuated confusion, not clarity.

The 1992 National Mental Health Reform Strategy had broad aspirations and called for reporting on areas of consumer and carer rights, legislation and other matters. Unable to meet the challenge of this breadth, initial reporting focused on the regular publication of mostly public mental health service activity data and related issues, such as expenditure and staffing. Some resources were provided initially to support the reporting process, but these were discontinued. This limited the further expansion of the reporting process.

As new plans emerged, the focus of mental health reforms shifted, seeking to consider issues beyond the health system. Since the CoAG in 2006, the reporting process has been subject to increasing pressure as competing policies and plans frequently emerged.

The initial clarity of purpose became confused. Commitments to better accountability were made, but resources were not provided. Mental health reporting has been managed and proceeded largely unchanged under MHISSC, leaving other mental health stakeholders outside the design process. All these factors have contributed to making the mental health data collection and reporting process less relevant over time.

Other existing mental health reporting mechanisms provided by the AIHW and the Productivity Commission focus on health services and operate without set targets. Neither impels identifiable processes of quality improvement. The new National Cabinet reporting arrangements established under COVID have diminished the mental health accountability obligations of all governments.

In 2020, the AIHW sought stakeholder views regarding a future National Health Information Strategy, considering issues such as data collection, access, reporting, privacy and so on, but without specific reference to mental health data. In response, some stakeholders suggested an urgent need for patient-reported outcome measures in mental health [68]. Mental Health Australia, the peak body, did not provide a submission to the AIHW. The separation of mental health data development from the rest of health has been a defining feature of the past thirty years of Australia's mental health strategy. There are clearly risks that this unhelpful separation could continue.

As of early 2022, the Australian government has been announcing a series of bilateral agreements with each of the eight states and territories which will form the backbone of the sixth National Mental Health and Suicide Prevention Plan [69]. Details of these arrangements, including data collection and reporting obligations, are yet to be made public.

The establishment of an entirely new accountability framework was a key recommendation of the Productivity Commission [46]. This framework will need to facilitate new approaches to regional modelling, governance and reporting across the whole 'ecosystem' of mental health. It will require expertise and resources. It must be based on a robust process of co-design, properly accounting for the different, but related, needs of planners, funders, service providers, consumers, carers, researchers and others. These are the ingredients for effective systemic oversight and local quality improvement. Such a system can build new community trust in our mental health system.

Author Contributions: S.R. prepared the manuscript of this article. L.S.-C., G.M. and I.H. provided comments and edited the paper. All authors have read and agreed to the published version of the manuscript.

Funding: This research received no external funding.

Conflicts of Interest: The authors declare no conflict of interest.

Appendix A

Table A1. Mental health data and accountability timeline.

Year	Policy Document	Notes in Relation to Data/Accountability
1992	First National Mental Health Strategy (and Policy)	
1993–1998	First National Mental Health Plan	Eight areas identified
1994	First National Mental Health Report	Established baseline
1995–2013	National Mental Health Report Series—11 editions	In 2013, 24 national indicators plus 18 indicators reported at jurisdictional level
1995	First Report on Government Services (ROGS) by Productivity Commission	2021 edition includes 60 tables of information (most recent year reported is 2018–2019).
1997	Evaluation of the First National Mental Health Plan	
1998-2003	Second National Mental Health Plan	
2001	First Mental Health Services in Australia report published by the Australian Institute of Health and Welfare.	2021 edition includes 35 tables of information (most recent year reported is 2018–2019).
2001	International Mid-Term Review of the Second National Mental Health Plan	
2003	Evaluation of the Second National Mental Health Plan	
2003–2008	Third National Mental Health Plan	34 outcomes, 113 key directions.
2005	National Mental Health Report (9th)	Summary of 10 Years of the National Mental Health Reform Strategy
2005	First National Mental Health Performance Framework	
2006–2011	Council of Australian Governments' National Action Plan on Mental Health	12 progress measures
2008	Evaluation of the Third National Mental Health Plan	
2009	Second National Mental Health Policy	Replacing the original 1992 document.
2009–2014	Fourth National Mental Health Plan	
2009	National Advisory Council on Mental Health	Recommended changing accountability framework for mental health (not actioned).
2010	Fourth National Mental Health Plan Implementation Strategy	
2011	Fourth National Mental Health Plan Measurement Strategy	5 key areas, 27 indicators.
2012–2022	Council of Australian Governments' National Roadmap for Mental Health Reform	11 'performance' indicators and 3 'contextual' indicators.
2012	National Mental Health First Report Card—A Contributing Life	Seven key areas reported.

Table A1. *Cont.*

Year	Policy Document	Notes in Relation to Data/Accountability
2014	National Mental Health Commission Review—Contributing Lives, Thriving Communities	Eight key indicators/targets identified for new reporting framework (not actioned).
2015	Australian Government Response to National Commission Review	Undertaken to develop new indicators as part of 5th National Mental Health Plan
2017	5th National Mental Health and Suicide Prevention Plan	24 indicators focusing on quality and safety
2020	Productivity Commission Report into Mental Health	6 key areas with 47 indicators recommended
2020	National mental health and wellbeing pandemic response plan	[Committed] to data collection and modelling, and the development of indicators for informed policy development
2020	CoAG process disbanded in favour of National Cabinet	
2021	Victorian Royal Commission into mental health	Recommended establishment of new regional mental health indicators under a Mental Health and Wellbeing Outcomes Framework
2021	Prevention, Compassion, Care—National Mental Health and Suicide Prevention Plan	Committed to developing new a National Agreement on Mental Health and Suicide Prevention between all governments.

References

1. Commonwealth Department of Human Services and Health. *National Mental Health Policy*; Commonwealth of Australia: Canberra, Australia, 1992.
2. Department of Prime Minister and Cabinet. COAG Becomes National Cabinet. Available online: https://www.pmc.gov.au/news-centre/government/coag-becomes-national-cabinet (accessed on 12 March 2022).
3. Mendoza, J.; Elson, A.; Gilbert, Y.; Bresnan, A.; Rosenberg, S.; Long, P.; Wilson, K.; Hopkins, J. *Obsessive Hope Disorder: Reflections on 30 Years of Mental Health Reform in Australia and Visions for the Future*; BJN Graphic Design: Caloundra, Australia, 2013.
4. Green, B.N.; Johnson, C.D.; Adams, A. Writing narrative literature reviews for peer-reviewed journals: Secrets of the trade. *J. Chiropr. Med.* **2006**, *5*, 101–117. [CrossRef]
5. Mulgan, R. Accountability: An ever-expanding concept? *Public Adm.* **2000**, *78*, 555–573. [CrossRef]
6. Eagar, K. ABF Information Series No. 1, What Is Activity-Based Funding? Available online: https://ro.uow.edu.au/cgi/viewcontent.cgi?referer=&httpsredir=1&article=1049&context=gsbpapers (accessed on 28 September 2021).
7. Moreno, K.; Sanchez, E.; Salvador-Carulla, L. Methodological Advances in Unit Cost Calculation of Psychiatric Residential Care in Spain. *J. Ment. Health Policy Econ.* **2008**, *11*, 79–88. [PubMed]
8. Institute of Medicine. *Improving the Quality of Health Care for Mental and Substance-Abuse Conditions*; National Academies Press: Washington, DC, USA, 2006.
9. Jenkins, R. Towards a system of outcome indicators for mental health care. *Br. J. Psychiatry* **1990**, *157*, 500–514. [CrossRef] [PubMed]
10. Brinkerhoff, D. *Accountability and Health Systems: Overview, Framework, and Strategies*; The Partners for Health Reform Plus Project; Abt Associates Inc Bethesda: Rockville, MD, USA, 2003.
11. Australian Institute of Health and Welfare. Mental Health Information Strategy Standing Committee. Available online: https://www.aihw.gov.au/reports/mental-health-services/mental-health-services-in-australia/national-mental-health-committees/mental-health-information-strategy-standing-committee (accessed on 28 September 2021).
12. Australian Institute of Health and Welfare; Australian Health Ministers' Advisory Council; National Health Information Management Group Australia. *National Health Information Agreement Procedure Manual*; Australian Institute of Health & Welfare: Canberra, Australia, 1994.

13. Department of Health and Ageing. *Tracking Progress of Mental Health Reform in Australia 1993–2011: National Mental Health Report 2013*; Commonwealth of Australia: Canberra, Australia, 2013.
14. Department of Human Services and Health. *National Mental Health Report 1994*; Australian Government Publishing Service: Canberra, Australia, 1995.
15. Australian Institute of Health and Welfare. National Minimum Data Sets and Data Set Specifications. Available online: https://meteor.aihw.gov.au/content/index.phtml/itemId/344846 (accessed on 28 September 2021).
16. Mental Health Council of Australia. *Measuring a Contributing Life*; Submission to the National Mental Health Commission: Canberra, Australia, 2013.
17. Smullen, A. Not Centralisation but Decentralised Integration through Australia's National Mental Health Policy. *Aust. J. Public Adm.* **2016**, *75*, 280–290. [CrossRef]
18. Australian Institute of Health and Welfare. Mental Health Services in Australia. Available online: https://www.aihw.gov.au/reports/mental-health-services/mhsa/national-mental-health-committees/mental-health-information-strategy-standing-commit (accessed on 24 January 2022).
19. National Mental Health Strategy Evaluation Steering Committee, for the Australian Health Ministers Advisory Council. *Evaluation of the National Mental Health Strategy: Final Report, Mental Health Branch*; Commonwealth Department of Health and Family Services: Canberra, Australia, 1997.
20. Whiteford, H. The Australian Health Ministers' Advisory Council (AHMAC) and the National Mental Health Reforms. *Australas. Psychiatry* **1994**, *2*, 101–104. [CrossRef]
21. Whiteford, H. Shaping Mental Health Policy in Australia 1988–2008. Ph.D. Thesis, Australian National University, Canberra, Australia, 29 July 2013.
22. Curie, C.; Thornicroft, G. *Summative Evaluation of the National Mental Health Plan 2003–2008*; Commonwealth of Australia: Canberra, Australia, 2008.
23. Australian Senate. *From Crisis to Community*; Select Committee on Mental Health: Canberra, Australia, 2006.
24. National Advisory Council on Mental Health. A Mentally Health Future for all Australians. November 2009. Available online: https://www.agac.org.au/assets/images/MentallyHealthyDisPap_200110.pdf (accessed on 11 March 2022).
25. Mental Health Council of Australia and the Australian Human Rights Commission. *Not For Service: Experiences of Injustice and Despair in Mental Health Care in Australia*; Mental Health Council of Australia: Canberra, Australia, 2005.
26. Australian Policy Observatory. National Action Plan on Mental Health 2006–2011; Council of Australian Governments (CoAG). Available online: https://apo.org.au/node/159056 (accessed on 28 September 2021).
27. Standing Council on Health. National Action Plan on Mental Health 2006–2011: Final Progress Report; Council of Australian Governments (CoAG): June 2013. Available online: https://studylib.net/doc/6755883/national-action-plan-for-mental-health-2006-2011 (accessed on 29 September 2021).
28. National Health and Hospital Reform Commission. *Beyond the Blame Game*; Australian Government: Canberra, Australia, 2008.
29. Bridgman, P.; Davis, G. What use is a policy cycle? Plenty, if the aim is clear. *Aust. J. Public Adm.* **2003**, *62*, 98–102. [CrossRef]
30. Department of Health. Release of the Roadmap for National Mental Health Reform. Available online: https://www1.health.gov.au/internet/publications/publishing.nsf/Content/suicide-prevention-activities-evaluation~{}background~{}release-of-roadmap (accessed on 29 September 2021).
31. Commonwealth of Australia. Fourth National Mental Health Plan Measurement Strategy. 2011. Available online: https://www.aihw.gov.au/getmedia/d8e52c84-a53f-4eef-a7e6-f81a5af94764/Fourth-national-mental-health-plan-measurement-strategy-2011.pdf.aspx (accessed on 11 March 2022).
32. Department of Health. The Fourth National Mental Health Plan. Available online: https://www1.health.gov.au/internet/publications/publishing.nsf/Content/mental-pubs-f-plan09-toc~{}mental-pubs-f-plan09-pla (accessed on 28 September 2021).
33. Australian Government. National Mental Health Commission: National Reports. Available online: https://www.mentalhealthcommission.gov.au/monitoring-and-reporting/national-reports (accessed on 29 September 2021).
34. National Mental Health Commission. *The National Review of Mental Health Programmes and Services*; NMHC: Sydney, Australia, 2014.
35. NSW Mental Health Commission. *Living Well: A Strategic Plan for Mental Health in NSW*; NSW Mental Health Commission: Sydney, Australia, 2012.
36. CoAG Health Council. The Fifth National Mental Health and Suicide Prevention Plan. Available online: https://www.mentalhealthcommission.gov.au/getmedia/0209d27b-1873-4245-b6e5-49e770084b81/Fifth-National-Mental-Health-and-Suicide-Prevention-Plan (accessed on 29 September 2021).
37. CoAG Health Council. The Fifth National Mental Health and Suicide Prevention Plan—Implementation Plan. Available online: https://www.mentalhealthcommission.gov.au/getmedia/7641fccf-4338-47a1-83af-f94c73d0aac2/Fifth-National-Mental-Health-and-Suicide-Prevention-Plan_Implementation-Plan (accessed on 29 September 2021).
38. Sadeniemi, M.; Almeda, N.; Salinas-Pérez, J.A.; Gutiérrez-Colosía, M.R.; García-Alonso, C.; Ala-Nikkola, T.; Joffe, G.; Pirkola, S.; Wahlbeck, K.; Cid, J.; et al. A comparison of mental health care systems in Northern and Southern Europe: A service mapping study. *Int. J. Environ. Res. Public Health* **2018**, *15*, 1133. [CrossRef] [PubMed]
39. Castelpietra, G.; Salvador-Carulla, L.; Almborg, A.H.; Fernandez, A.; Madden, R. Working draft: Classifications of interventions in mental health care: An expert review. *Eur. J. Psychiatry* **2017**, *31*, 127–144. [CrossRef]

40. Crosbie, D.W. Mental health policy—Stumbling in the dark? *Med. J. Australia.* **2009**, *190*, S43–S45. [CrossRef] [PubMed]
41. Australian Institute of Health and Welfare. Mental Health Indicator Library. Available online: https://www.aihw.gov.au/reports/mental-health-services/mental-health-services-in-australia/report-contents/mental-health-indicators/mental-health-indicator-library (accessed on 29 September 2021).
42. Australian Institute of Health and Welfare. Mental Health Services Key Performance Indicators. Available online: https://www.aihw.gov.au/getmedia/245cf334-e277-4948-9449-67190f3bdde0/Mental-health-service-key-performance-indicators-tables.xlsx.aspx (accessed on 29 September 2021).
43. Australian Institute of Health and Welfare. National Mental Health Performance Framework. Available online: https://www.aihw.gov.au/getmedia/34959bca-4bb3-4229-a276-d6012e115687/National-Mental-Health-Performance-Framework-002.docx.aspx (accessed on 29 September 2021).
44. Productivity Commission. Report on Government Services, Chapter 13. Available online: https://www.pc.gov.au/research/ongoing/report-on-government-services/2021/health/services-for-mental-health (accessed on 29 September 2021).
45. McGuire, L.; Prior Jonson, E.; Perryman, S.; McKeown, T. Benchmarking government: Report on government services (RoGS)–25 years on. *Aust. J. Public Adm.* **2021**, *80*, 987–1001. [CrossRef]
46. Productivity Commission. *Mental Health, Report No. 95*; Commonwealth of Australia: Canberra, Australia, 2020.
47. State of Victoria. *Royal Commission into Victoria's Mental Health System, Final Report, Summary and Recommendations*; Parl Paper No. 202, Session 2018-21; The Royal Commission into Victoria's Mental Health System: Melbourne, Australia, 2021.
48. Productivity Commission. National Performance Reporting Dashboard. Available online: https://performancedashboard.d61.io/healthcare (accessed on 29 September 2021).
49. Australian Government. Prevention, Compassion, Care: National Mental Health and Suicide Prevention Plan. Available online: https://www.health.gov.au/sites/default/files/documents/2021/05/the-australian-government-s-national-mental-health-and-suicide-prevention-plan-national-mental-health-and-suicide-prevention-plan.pdf (accessed on 29 September 2021).
50. Primary Health Insights. Available online: https://www.primaryhealthinsights.org.au/ (accessed on 29 September 2021).
51. Department of Health. Primary Mental Health Care Data Set. Available online: https://pmhc-mds.com/#:~{}:text=The%20Primary%20Mental%20Health%20Care%20Minimum%20Data%20Set,health%20care%20services%20funded%20by%20the%20Australian%20Government (accessed on 29 September 2021).
52. Furst, M.A.; Bagheri, N.; Salvador-Carulla, L. An ecosystems approach to mental health services research. *BJPsych Int.* **2021**, *18*, 23–25. [CrossRef] [PubMed]
53. Rosenberg, S.; Rosen, A. It's raining mental health commissions: Prospects and pitfalls in driving mental health reform. *Australas. Psychiatry* **2012**, *20*, 85–90. [CrossRef] [PubMed]
54. AHMAC and Mental Health Information Strategy Subcommittee. *National Mental Health Benchmarking Project Evaluation Report, MHISS Discussion Paper No. 7*; Commonwealth of Australia: Canberra, Australia, 2009.
55. Australian Institute of Health and Welfare. Medicare Subsidised Services. Available online: https://www.aihw.gov.au/reports/mental-health-services/mental-health-services-in-australia/report-contents/medicare-subsidised-services (accessed on 28 September 2021).
56. Zabell, T.; Long, K.M.; Scott, D.; Hope, J.; McLoughlin, I.; Enticott, J. Engaging Healthcare Staff and Stakeholders in Healthcare Simulation Modeling for Research Translation: A Systematic Review. *Front. Health Serv.* **2021**, *1*, 3. [CrossRef]
57. Buckingham, B. Witness Statement to Victorian Royal Commission into Mental Health. Available online: http://rcvmhs.archive.royalcommission.vic.gov.au/Buckingham_Bill.pdf (accessed on 29 September 2021).
58. National Mental Health and Consumer Care Forum Advocacy Brief. Co-Design and Co-Production. Available online: http://nmhccf.org.au/sites/default/files/docs/nmhccf_-_co-design_and_co-production_ab_-_final_-_october_2017_0.pdf (accessed on 29 September 2021).
59. Slade, M.; Leese, M.; Cahill, S.; Thornicroft, G.; Kuipers, E. Patient-rated mental health needs and quality of life improvement. *Br. J. Psychiatry* **2005**, *187*, 256–261. [CrossRef] [PubMed]
60. Hickie, I.B.; Davenport, T.A.; Burns, J.M.; Milton, A.C.; Ospina-Pinillos, L.; Whittle, L.; Ricci, C.S.; McLoughlin, L.T.; Mendoza, J.; Cross, S.P.; et al. Project Synergy: Co-designing technology-enabled solutions for Australian mental health services reform. *Med. J. Aust.* **2019**, *211*, S3–S39. [CrossRef] [PubMed]
61. Mārama, T.P. Real-Time Feedback. Available online: https://www.tepou.co.nz/initiatives/marama-real-time-feedback (accessed on 29 September 2021).
62. Australian Institute of Health and Welfare. Your Experience of Care Survey. Available online: https://www.aihw.gov.au/reports/mental-health-services/mental-health-services-in-australia/national-mental-health-committees/mental-health-information-strategy-standing-committee/your-experience-of-service-survey-instrument (accessed on 29 September 2021).
63. Wong, Y.C.; Davis, A.; Hudson, P.; Wright, E.; Leitch, E.; Allan, J. National Mental Health Service Planning Framework-Implementation of joined-up regional planning of mental health service delivery. *Int. J. Integr. Care* **2018**, *18*, 1. [CrossRef]
64. García-Alonso, C.R.; Almeda, N.; Salinas-Pérez, J.A.; Gutiérrez-Colosía, M.R.; Uriarte-Uriarte, J.J.; Salvador-Carulla, L. A decision support system for assessing management interventions in a mental health ecosystem: The case of Bizkaia (Basque Country, Spain). *PLoS ONE* **2019**, *14*, e0212179. [CrossRef] [PubMed]
65. Atkinson, J.A.; Skinner, A.; Lawson, K.; Rosenberg, S.; Hickie, I.B. Bringing new tools, a regional focus, resource-sensitivity, local engagement and necessary discipline to mental health policy and planning. *BMC Public Health* **2020**, *20*, 814. [CrossRef] [PubMed]

66. Organisation for Economic Cooperation and Development. A New Benchmark for Mental Health Systems. Available online: https://www.oecd.org/health/a-new-benchmark-for-mental-health-systems-4ed890f6-en.htm (accessed on 3 April 2022).
67. WHO European Framework for Action on Mental Health 2021–2025. Available online: https://apps.who.int/iris/bitstream/handle/10665/344609/WHO-EURO-2021-3147-42905-59865-eng.pdf?sequence=1&isAllowed=y (accessed on 3 April 2022).
68. Royal Australian College of General Practice (RACGP). Submission on AIHW's National Health Information Strategy Draft Framework. Available online: https://www.racgp.org.au/FSDEDEV/media/documents/RACGP/Reports%20and%20submissions/2020/RACGP-response-to-AIHW-on-NHIS-draft-framework-March-2020.pdf (accessed on 24 January 2022).
69. Hunt, G. Landmark Agreement Begins a New Era for Mental Health Care in NSW. Available online: https://www.health.gov.au/ministers/the-hon-greg-hunt-mp/media/landmark-agreement-begins-a-new-era-for-mental-health-care-in-nsw (accessed on 11 March 2022).

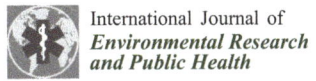

International Journal of *Environmental Research and Public Health*

Brief Report

Mental Health Services Data Dashboards for Reporting to Australian Governments during COVID-19

Sonam Shelly, Emily Lodge, Carly Heyman, Felicity Summers *, Amy Young, Jennifer Brew and Matthew James

Australian Institute of Health and Welfare, Canberra 2617, Australia; sonam.shelly@aihw.gov.au (S.S.); emily.lodge@aihw.gov.au (E.L.); carly.heyman@aihw.gov.au (C.H.); amy.young@aihw.gov.au (A.Y.); jennifer.brew@aihw.gov.au (J.B.); matthew.james@aihw.gov.au (M.J.)
* Correspondence: felicity.summers@aihw.gov.au

Abstract: The Australian Institute of Health and Welfare (AIHW) has been providing support to the Australian Government Department of Health to report on mental health-related data to Australian governments on a frequent basis since April 2020 in the form of COVID-19 mental health services data dashboards. These dashboards feature extensive use of data visualizations which illustrate the change in mental health service use over time as well as comparisons with pre-pandemic levels of service use. Data are included from the Medicare Benefits Schedule (MBS), Pharmaceutical Benefits Scheme (PBS/RPBS), Australian Government-funded crisis and support organizations, and key findings from emerging research. Demand for telehealth, crisis and support organizations and online mental health information services, in particular, have increased during the pandemic. The dashboards incorporate both new and existing data sources and represent an innovative way of reporting mental health services data to Australian governments. The reporting has enabled timely, targeted adjustments to mental health service delivery during the pandemic with improved cooperative data sharing arrangements having the potential to yield ongoing benefits.

Citation: Shelly, S.; Lodge, E.; Heyman, C.; Summers, F.; Young, A.; Brew, J.; James, M. Mental Health Services Data Dashboards for Reporting to Australian Governments during COVID-19. *Int. J. Environ. Res. Public Health* **2021**, *18*, 10514. https://doi.org/10.3390/ijerph181910514

Academic Editor: Richard Madden

Received: 3 September 2021
Accepted: 30 September 2021
Published: 7 October 2021

Publisher's Note: MDPI stays neutral with regard to jurisdictional claims in published maps and institutional affiliations.

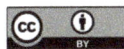

Copyright: © 2021 by the authors. Licensee MDPI, Basel, Switzerland. This article is an open access article distributed under the terms and conditions of the Creative Commons Attribution (CC BY) license (https://creativecommons.org/licenses/by/4.0/).

Keywords: mental; services; pandemic; COVID-19

1. Introduction

The global impact of the COVID-19 pandemic on mental health and wellbeing has been significant. The potential for this impact was recognized early in the pandemic and includes the direct health impacts of COVID-19 and fear of contagion, as well as the broader social and economic disruption [1].

In the Australian context, despite having experienced some significant COVID-19 outbreaks, containment measures have meant that the epidemic to date (July 2021) has generally been less severe than in many countries. However, the social, economic and mental health and wellbeing impacts of restrictions have been significant. Social distancing, sudden and protracted 'lockdowns', interruption of physical and mental health service provision, loss of employment, restricted international travel and border quarantine, and remote school and work have all had significant consequences. The impact of the pandemic in Australia started directly after an extreme drought and bushfire season for the country, a time of heightened anxiety for much of the population [2]. Data about the mental health effects of the pandemic at a national and international level are still evolving.

The Australian Institute of Health and Welfare (AIHW) has a long history in reporting mental health data, particularly through the Mental Health Services in Australia report and more recently the National Suicide and Self-harm Monitoring Project, a collaboration between the AIHW, the National Mental Health Commission and the Australian Government Department of Health (DoH), funded by the DoH. One of the key goals of this project is to improve the timeliness of state and territory data on suspected deaths by suicide.

A range of Australian research and reporting has been taking place on the mental health impacts of COVID-19 since early 2020. Some significant efforts include the Australian

National University's COVID-19 Impact Monitoring Survey Program, a longitudinal survey for which the AIHW provides financial support. This project seeks to monitor the economic and social wellbeing impacts of COVID-19 and is conducted through the ANUPoll, an ongoing quarterly probability-based panel survey of Australian public opinion. The availability of longitudinal pre-pandemic data from the ANUPoll facilitates analysis of the factors that have contributed to pandemic driven changes in psychological distress. The Australian Bureau of Statistics (ABS) has also been conducting surveys to investigate the impacts of the COVID-19 pandemic. From April 2020 to June 2021, the monthly Household Impacts of COVID-19 Survey collected longitudinal data on a range of topics including psychological distress. The Melbourne Institute (University of Melbourne) also commenced the Taking the Pulse of the Nation survey in April 2020.

Data were collected on a broad range of measures of mental health and wellbeing during the pandemic in Australia, including suicide and self-harm [3], life satisfaction, anxiety and worry [4], social connection, personal stressors, self-reported mental health [5] and use of mental health services [6]. One particularly relevant measure to the utilization of mental health services is that of psychological distress, commonly measured using the Kessler Psychological Distress Scale. A higher proportion of Australians have reported severe psychological distress during than pre-pandemic. Psychological distress and related measures tended to show peaks early in the pandemic and in conjunction with lockdowns, with elevated levels around April 2020 and again around August to October 2020 [4,5], the latter peak likely reflecting the impact of the relatively severe second wave in Victoria.

There was significant concern early in the pandemic about its potential impact on deaths by suicide [7], in part based on research linking unemployment to increased suicide rates [8]. Data on suspected deaths by suicide in 2020 for three Australian state suicide registers are included in the National Suicide and Self-harm Monitoring Project. This project seeks to improve the understanding of suicide and self-harm in Australia, to help identify factors that increase risk, to raise awareness and improve support and prevention activities. The AIHW routinely receives data for some states and territories, which is included in the dashboards. A key aim of the project is to establish registers for all Australian states and territories. To date, there has not been evidence of an increase in suspected deaths by suicide in any of these jurisdictions compared to previous years, however, the situation is complex and it remains important to continue to monitor the impact on suicide risk over time [3].

Analysis of ambulance attendances (one month per quarter data snapshots) available for some Australian states and territories from the National Ambulance Surveillance System (part of the National Suicide and Self-harm Monitoring Project) showed slight spikes in the population rate of ambulance attendances for self-injury and suicidal ideation during the outbreak period of the September 2020 quarter in Victoria. There was also a gradual increase in both measures between December 2019 and December 2020, particularly self-injury (4.7 to 6.5 per 100,000 population), although the rate of attendances for suicide attempts fell from 14.9 to 12.4 in the state over that year. Gradual increases in the rate of attendances for self-injury were also evident in the Australian Capital Territory (6.8 to 10.0) and Tasmania (2.1 to 5.9) over the period [9], however, whether these changes were related to the pandemic is unclear.

The impacts of the pandemic have not been evenly experienced across the Australian population. People with pre-existing mental health conditions [2] and few social supports [1] are at increased risk of distress. In general, younger Australians [10] and women have tended to have worse mental health outcomes than other Australians during the pandemic. Among young people (aged 44 and under), average psychological distress scores were elevated in 2020 compared to 2017, with the greatest increases for those aged 18–24 years. Women and people living in Victoria were the main drivers of an increase in psychological distress from May to August 2020 [11]. High mental distress (defined as 'feeling depressed' and/or 'anxious' 'most or all of the time') among parents also increased, from 8% in 2017 to 24% in 2020 [12].

There is evidence that the economic downturn associated with the pandemic has increased levels of psychological distress, with those employed in April 2020 having significantly lower levels of psychological distress than the unemployed at that time, when considering only those employed in February 2020 [13]. Rates of mental distress were approximately four times higher for people experiencing financial stress (42%) compared to people not experiencing financial distress (11.5%) during April to November 2020 [12].

The OECD has identified a similar range of increased risk factors associated with the pandemic which have contributed to a worsening of mental health, including unemployment and financial insecurity, reduced social connections, difficulties associated with telework, home schooling and education, restricted exercise and reduced access to health services. Peaks of mental distress have been closely related to waves of COVID-19 cases when restrictions have been most stringent [14]. The use of data visualizations in recent OECD reporting clearly illustrates some of the mental health impacts of COVID-19 across nations, particularly regarding depression and anxiety both during the pandemic and in comparison to pre-pandemic periods [14].

The mental health services system in Australia is complex and varies by state and territory, with some services funded by the Australian Government, others by state and territory governments or both. Mental health services are provided through public and private hospitals, residential and community mental health care, by specialist psychiatric and general medical practitioners, mental health nurses, psychologists and other allied health professionals. There are a range of crisis support services, as well as services provided through the National Disability Insurance Scheme and the non-government sector [15]. Australia's federated model of health care also means that there is no single 'master' data set relating to health services.

Due to the complexity of the Australian mental health system and the need for timely data collection and analysis to guide the provision of mental health services during the pandemic [16], the AIHW has been providing support to the DoH to report on mental health-related data to Australian governments since April 2020, funded by the DoH. The COVID-19 National Mental Health Services dashboard and later the State and Territory Mental Health Services dashboard, were produced weekly during 2020, and fortnightly in 2021. These reports provide summary statistics of recent data and comparisons with the same data from early and pre-pandemic periods and extensive use of data visualizations of change over time. Data sources include information from the Medicare Benefits Schedule (MBS), Pharmaceutical Benefits Scheme (PBS) and Repatriation Pharmaceutical Benefits Scheme (RPBS), Australian Government-funded crisis and support organizations, and a brief summary of emerging research. A publicly available summary of the data is reported in the AIHW online publication, Mental Health Services in Australia [6], updated quarterly.

The aim of the present paper is to describe the background, development process, key results and learnings from the compilation of the data for the National Mental Health Services and State and Territory Mental Health Services dashboards. The processes that have led to success, and improvements in communication and data sharing within and across government and non-government organizations have broader implications for future health data, information and policy development.

2. Materials and Methods

2.1. Environment Scan

An environment scan and literature review were conducted to determine the range of Australian research and data holdings that were being established in relation to COVID-19 and mental health. During the initial scoping for the dashboard reporting, it was recognized that some of the organizations that would first see the impact of the pandemic on service utilization were those for which there was no national data collection, in particular, crisis and support organizations and online mental health information services.

2.2. Data Sources

2.2.1. Crisis and Support Organizations and Online Mental Health Information Services

There are a number of Australian phone and online crisis and support services available to people seeking support for mental health issues. Crisis and support organization data include call, web chat, 'app' use, online programs and forums, and/or email data from a range of organizations, including Lifeline, Kids Helpline, Beyond Blue, Smiling Mind's Healthcare Worker Program, Head to Health, Black Dog Institute and ReachOut. Data for HeadtoHelp hubs (Victorian Mental Health Clinics) also include face-to-face contacts.

2.2.2. Medicare Benefits Schedule and Pharmaceutical Benefits Scheme Data

Services Australia collects fee-for-service related MBS claims activity data which it supplies to the DoH [17]. The Australian Government introduced additional MBS telehealth items during the COVID-19 pandemic, including items for mental health services provided by psychiatrists, GPs, allied health professionals and psychologists. MBS subsidized services under the Better Access to Psychiatrists, Psychologists and General Practitioners through the MBS (Better Access) initiative were also expanded [18]. MBS data reported in the dashboards include use of MBS mental health items (services processed), the proportion of services delivered via telehealth, and MBS benefits paid.

The Australian Government subsidizes the cost of prescription medicines through two schemes, the PBS and RPBS for eligible veterans and their dependents. Services Australia processes all prescriptions dispensed under the PBS/RPBS and provides these data to the DoH [19]. PBS/RPBS data reported includes the number of PBS dispensed mental health-related prescriptions.

Further information on these data sources is available at https://www.aihw.gov.au/reports/mental-health-services/mental-health-services-in-australia/ (accessed on 5 October 2021).

2.2.3. Emerging Research

Key points from emerging research are provided in each dashboard update, with a more detailed discussion in the Mental Health Services in Australia quarterly online update. This includes key findings from research programs outlined in the introduction to this article.

2.3. Data Access and Analysis

2.3.1. Data Access and Metric Selection

The data supply from crisis and support organizations and online mental health information services to the AIHW was established in collaboration with the DoH, facilitated through their existing contractual arrangements with the agencies. A prototype data collection template was prepared by the AIHW, with adjustments made as required for individual agency collections. The collection includes daily data on contact volumes and weekly aggregate data on some demographic variables including age, sex, Indigenous status, state or territory and reason for call. Due to data quality issues, reporting of demographic variables (particularly Indigenous status and age) has been limited.

Under an existing arrangement with the DoH, the AIHW had access to the MBS and PBS/RPBS data via the Department's Enterprise Data Warehouse (EDW) for use in AIHW's regular reporting products. A list of MBS item numbers relating to mental health was identified, based largely on the AIHW's existing Mental health services in Australia reporting. Early analysis identified key metrics for reporting, which have been refined over time. Mental health-related prescriptions in the PBS/RPBS data were identified using Anatomic Therapeutic Chemical (ATC) codes and ongoing trend analysis included from November 2020.

The dashboard was initially funded and prepared for a national view of mental health impacts. Clear gaps became evident early in the process, significantly that the dashboard only included data from Australian Government funded services; it was missing data from the public mental health system run by state and territory governments. In addition, situations in each state and territory have varied markedly, with the majority of cases occurring in two states, Victoria and New South Wales. On behalf of the DoH, the AIHW established processes to share data across levels of government and developed an agreement to include data at the state and territory level. Data sharing initially focused on the two most populous states of New South Wales and Victoria (together comprising 58% of the total population) which had the largest COVID-19 case numbers (87% of all cases to April 2021) [20]. Agreements were established by the AIHW on behalf of the DoH, for participating states to provide emergency department, community mental health care services and admitted patient (hospitals) data at the required intervals, with the AIHW providing MBS and crisis and support organization data back to these states for their own reporting and monitoring purposes. Queensland subsequently joined the data sharing arrangement and was included in the State and Territory Mental Health Services dashboard from May 2021. Data for Queensland will be included in AIHW's reporting on Mental health service in Australia from October 2021.

2.3.2. Data Analysis

Data were analysed in SAS Enterprise Guide 7.1 and Microsoft Excel©. Data visualizations were created in Tableau software version 2020.3. The data were presented as A3 colour posters, with data and graphics grouped by data source.

There are hundreds of mental health-related MBS items, and items are often added and removed from the schedule. The list of items analysed were similar to that described in Mental health services in Australia [21]. MBS data were analyzed by date of processing, as this results in more stable historical values over time. During code development, the extraction method was validated by reviewing results against those obtained through the Australian Government Services Australia Medicare Item Reports tool [22]. When extracting data, it was also ensured that data existed up to the last date of interest, to ensure that analyses were not impacted by unanticipated delays to data warehouse updates.

PBS items analyzed included antipsychotics (N05A), anxiolytics (N05B), hypnotics and sedatives (N05C), antidepressants (N06A), and psychostimulants, agents used for ADHD and nootropics (N06B), according to the Anatomical Therapeutic Chemical (ATC) Classification System [23]. PBS data were lagged by at least 6 weeks from the extraction date to reduce the effect of late claims, updates and cancellations.

Statistics supplied by non-government organizations were routinely checked for consistency with historical supplies. Any changes to historical values were queried with the supplying organization, and then corrected if necessary. Time series were also routinely inspected manually for any anomalies or unusual patterns, which were also queried. Furthermore, these organizations may run their own data cleansing procedures from time to time, resulting in minor changes to historical values.

3. Results

The following is a summary of the publicly available results for data to 25 April 2021 for the COVID-19 National Mental Health Services Dashboard and limited data from the state level dashboard, published in Mental Health Services in Australia in July 2021 [6]. In addition to data visualizations and descriptions of trends over time, the following descriptions include comparisons of the most recent publicly available (at time of writing) month of data compared with the same month in 2020 and 2019. These comparisons are provided in the dashboards to help illustrate differences between pre-pandemic, early pandemic and more recent data.

3.1. Use of Medicare-Subsidised Mental Health-Related Services

- MBS mental health service usage showed a generally upward trend from early April 2020 to end of April 2021, with temporary dips observed during major holiday periods. Over 15.0 million MBS-subsidized mental health-related services were delivered

- between 16 March 2020 and 25 April 2021, with just under one third (29.5%) delivered by telehealth. The number of services delivered in the 4 weeks to 25 April 2021, was almost one fifth higher than the number of services provided in the same 4-week period in 2020 and 2019.
- Delivery of MBS subsidized mental health services via telehealth peaked in April 2020, when about half of these services were delivered remotely, corresponding with Australia's national lockdown in April—May 2020 (Figure 1).

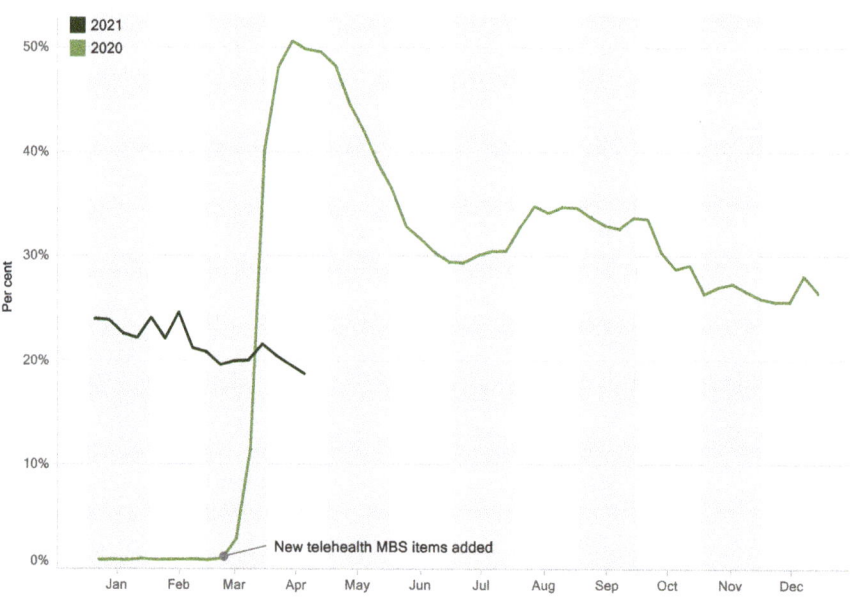

Figure 1. MBS mental health telehealth services (proportion of all MBS mental health services), January 2020–April 2021. (Website: https://www.aihw.gov.au/reports/mental-health-services/mental-health-services-in-australia/report-contents/covid-19-impact-on-mental-health, accessed on 5 October 2021).

3.2. Pharmaceutical Benefits Scheme (PBS) Prescriptions

- There was a spike in all mental health-related PBS-subsidized and under co-payment prescriptions in the 4 weeks to 29 March 2020 at the peak of Australia's initial outbreak, an 18.6% increase in the number of prescriptions dispensed compared to the same period in 2019 (Figure 2).

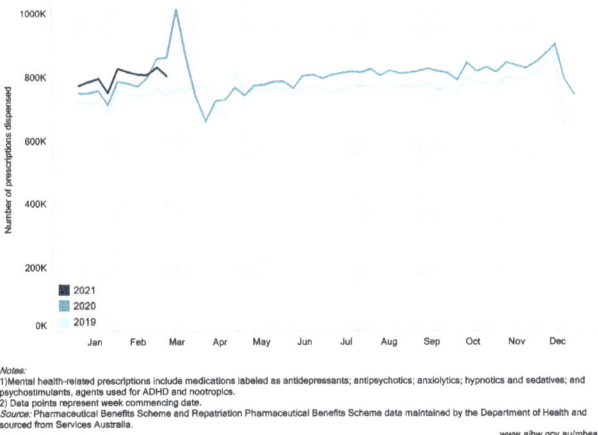

Figure 2. PBS mental health-related prescriptions dispensed (by week), January 2019–March 2021. (Website: https://www.aihw.gov.au/reports/mental-health-services/mental-health-services-in-australia/report-contents/covid-19-impact-on-mental-health, accessed on 5 October 2021).

3.3. Use of Crisis and Support Organisations and Online Mental Health Information Services

Crisis and support organizations and online mental health information services have reported significant demand increases during the pandemic. Calls to Lifeline increased in 2020 compared to 2019 and have stayed at an elevated level.

Contacts with Beyond Blue increased in March 2020 and stayed elevated throughout the year, settling into a level between 2019 and 2020 volumes in March—April 2021. Kids Helpline contacts spiked in early April 2020, and trended down over the course of 2020, settling back to 2019 levels in 2021 (Figure 3).

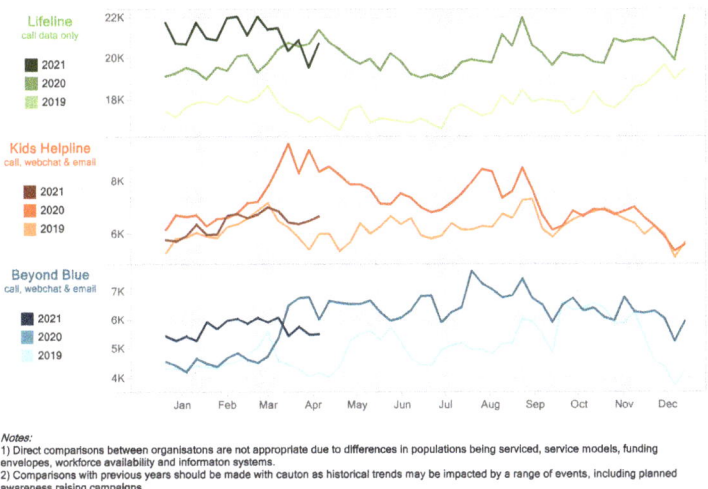

Figure 3. Crisis and support organization contacts (by week), January 2019–April 2021. (Website: https://www.aihw.gov.au/reports/mental-health-services/mental-health-services-in-australia/report-contents/covid-19-impact-on-mental-health, accessed on 5 October 2021).

In the 4 weeks to 25 April 2021 (compared to the same period in 2020 and 2019):
- Almost 82,000 calls were made to Lifeline, a similar volume (2.3% decrease) to April 2020 and an 18.4% increase from April 2019;
- Over 22,000 contacts were made with Beyond Blue, a 14.9% decrease and 30.7% increase from April 2020 and 2019, respectively;
- Approximately 26,000 contact attempts were made to Kids Helpline (not including those abandoned during the privacy message), a 26.6% decrease and 10.5% increase from April 2020 and 2019, respectively;
- Head to Health and ReachOut websites had an increase in visits at the start of the pandemic, with a peak in March 2020. ReachOut reported approximately 7600 daily website visits in April 2021, decreases of 34.5% and 13.2% compared to April 2020 and 2019, respectively. Head to Health reported about 1400 users per day in April 2021, a 74.7% decrease and 37.0% increase compared to the same periods in 2020 and 2019, respectively.

3.4. Jurisdictional Differences in Mental Health Service Activity

Data by some Australian states and territories is included in a state level dashboard, which is supplementary to the national dashboard. Publicly available reporting on this jurisdictional dashboard is currently only available for New South Wales and Victoria.

Australian states and territories have experienced varying levels of outbreaks over the course of the pandemic, striking at different time periods, ranging from no community transmission to the large 'second wave' outbreak in Victoria in winter 2020. Pandemic outbreaks and associated restrictions show clear patterns in the use of MBS telehealth services and use of crisis and support organizations.

- The population rate of MBS mental health services was generally higher throughout the course of 2020 than during 2019, in both states, with the differential most evident in Victoria from the second half of 2020 onwards. This elevated rate is still evident in 2021. This pattern was likely influenced by the introduction of 10 additional subsidized psychology sessions under the Better Access initiative to people living under lockdown initially, which was then expanded to all Australians.
- The 4 weeks to 13 September 2020 in Victoria and the 4 weeks to 7 March 2020 in New South Wales were the periods with the highest number of MBS mental health-related services with about 360,000 services in each state.
- In New South Wales, there was an initial steep increase in telehealth services between March and April 2020, followed by a gradual decline, consistent with the pattern for the country overall. Victoria showed a double peak in telehealth service use, consistent with the second wave in winter 2020, and a small but sharp spike in February 2021 at the time of a smaller outbreak in Victoria (Figure 4).
- There have been some clear jurisdictional differences since the beginning of the pandemic in the rate of crisis and support organization contacts. In Victoria, calls to Beyond Blue showed a notable spike, commencing in July 2020, consistent with the onset of their second wave. The rate of call volumes to Lifeline, Kids Helpline and Beyond Blue all showed a greater difference between 2019 and 2020 in Victoria than in New South Wales. However, Lifeline and Kids Helpline both showed a notable ongoing higher level of call volume in NSW in 2020 than in 2019. Lifeline calls in NSW in the early part of 2021 were notably higher, possibly related to the northern beaches outbreak at that time.

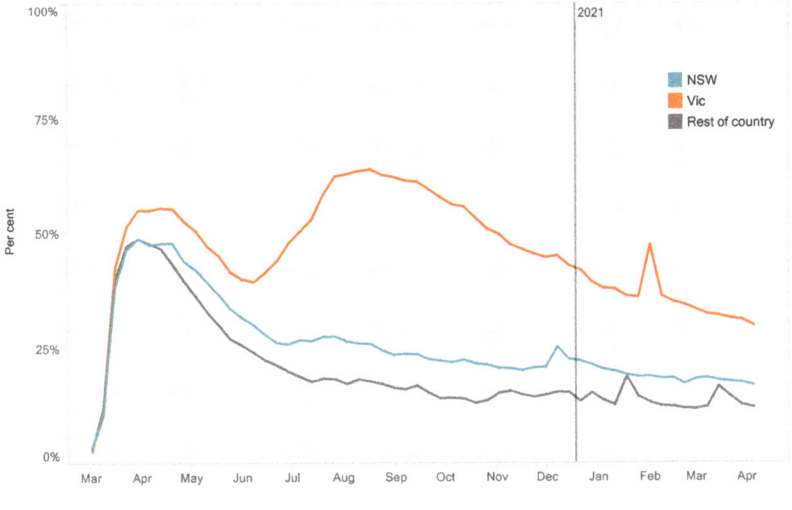

Figure 4. MBS mental health telehealth services (proportion of all MBS mental health services), by jurisdiction, March 2020–April 2021. (Website: https://www.aihw.gov.au/reports/mental-health-services/mental-health-services-in-australia/report-contents/covid-19-impact-on-mental-health, accessed on 5 October 2021).

4. Discussion

The COVID-19 mental health services dashboards represent an innovative way of reporting high level mental health services data to Australian governments.

Much of the data included in the dashboards had not been reported in this way previously, including data from crisis and support organizations and online mental health information services. The dashboards include a variety of data in one view, over time, at frequent reporting intervals, giving a unique overview and triangulation of data sources that lead to additional insights and confirmation of patterns in service demand and use. Interactions and common movements across different types of service use are readily visible, demonstrating clearly the impacts of the pandemic relative to baseline results, and the influence of lockdowns, other restrictions and outbreaks evident in service use over time. This has enabled the data to form an integral part of the evidence base drawn on by Australian governments to determine adjustments to mental health service provision during the pandemic.

The frequent reporting has supported ongoing, timely reporting improvement both through internal review and frequent feedback from external stakeholders. High frequency reporting has been far more informative than annual reporting could be in the current context.

Ongoing communication with and between data receivers, providers and the analysis team has been crucial when unexpected changes in the data have been observed, so as to avoid spurious conclusions. In some cases, changes in service use have been due to planned service delivery changes rather than pandemic related demand changes.

Maintaining agility and being alert to shifting trends in the data has been an ongoing challenge, particularly given the tight timeframes inherent in weekly and fortnightly reporting. Consideration is being given to the potential benefits of presenting the dashboard material as a restricted release online webpage in future, to allow greater interaction for end users and more flexibility in presentation of content.

As noted above, the present description of the dashboard results is limited to those publicly available at the time of writing. Ongoing updates to the data are published on a quarterly basis in the Mental health services in Australia online publication.

It should be noted that while reporting of aggregate data on mental health service use provides useful insights into the utilization of mental health services, it cannot provide information on either the adequacy of services or the benefits of treatment at the individual level. Neither should it be assumed that the pandemic is the underlying reason for all changes in mental health service use over the reporting period.

There is no 'master' data set for reporting on the use of mental health services in Australia. The data presented in the dashboards are limited to aspects of the mental health system for which adequate data are available or could be readily developed for reporting on a frequent (i.e., at least fortnightly) basis. The AIHW will continue to work to improve available data on the use of mental health services.

5. Conclusions

The reporting of data on mental health service use in Australia is evolving. While large administrative data sets are a valuable source of epidemiological data, traditionally long lead times have often limited their utility for governments responding to time sensitive issues. The use of administrative data to inform policy responses to emerging challenges, notably, disaster recovery and the impact of the COVID-19 pandemic, has required governments to adapt existing protocols, particularly relating to data timeframes, to meet these new needs.

The COVID-19 mental health services dashboard project and associated reporting has involved new levels of data sharing and communication between Australian and state and territory governments, and non-government organizations on the utilization of mental health services in Australia. The project has demonstrated willingness and ability of these organizations to implement cooperative data sharing arrangements that have the potential to lead to ongoing benefits that extend beyond the pandemic.

Author Contributions: Conceptualization, A.Y. and S.S.; methodology, A.Y. and S.S.; formal analysis, S.S., C.H., E.L. and J.B.; investigation, A.Y.; data curation, A.Y., S.S. and J.B.; writing—original draft preparation, F.S.; writing—review and editing, A.Y., S.S., M.J., C.H. and E.L.; visualization, S.S., C.H. and E.L. All authors have read and agreed to the published version of the manuscript.

Funding: Funding for this project is provided by the Australian Government Department of Health under the National Suicide and Self-harm Monitoring Project.

Institutional Review Board Statement: Not applicable.

Informed Consent Statement: Not applicable. Analyses involve anonymous administrative data.

Data Availability Statement: The de-identified unit record datasets used to generate the present analyses are not publicly available. Further data related to the mental health COVID-19 dashboards is available at https://www.aihw.gov.au/reports/mental-health-services/mental-health-services-in-australia/report-contents/mental-health-impact-of-COVID-19 (accessed on 5 October 2021).

Conflicts of Interest: The authors declare no conflict of interest.

References

1. WHO (World Health Organization). Substantial Investment Needed to Avert Mental Health Crisis. Available online: https://www.who.int/news/item/14-05-2020-substantial-investment-needed-to-avert-mental-health-crisis (accessed on 29 June 2021).
2. Black Dog Institute. *Mental Health Ramifications of COVD-19: The Australian Context*; Black Dog Institute: Sydney, Australia, 2020.
3. Australian Institute of Health and Welfare. Suicide and Self-Harm Monitoring. Available online: https://www.aihw.gov.au/suicide-self-harm-monitoring/data (accessed on 28 June 2021).
4. Biddle, N.; Gray, M. *Tracking Wellbeing Outcomes during the COVID-19 Pandemic (April 2021): Continued Social and Economic Recovery and Resilience*; Australian National University (ANU) Centre for Social Research Methods: Canberra, Australia, 2021.
5. Australian Bureau of Statistics. Household Impacts of COVID-19 Survey (April and May 2021). Available online: https://www.abs.gov.au/statistics/people/people-and-communities/household-impacts-covid-19-survey (accessed on 28 June 2021).

6. Australian Institute of Health and Welfare. Mental Health Services in Australia. Mental Health Impact of COVID-19. Available online: https://www.aihw.gov.au/reports/mental-health-services/mental-health-services-in-australia/report-contents/mental-health-impact-of-covid-19 (accessed on 28 June 2021).
7. Royal Australian College of General Practitioners. Sharp Suicide Increase Expected Due to Pandemic. Available online: https://www1.racgp.org.au/newsgp/clinical/calls-for-urgent-attention-to-covid-related-mental (accessed on 12 July 2021).
8. University of Sydney. Integrated Modelling Pre-Empts Friday's National Cabinet Meeting. Available online: https://www.sydney.edu.au/news-opinion/news/2020/05/13/modelling-shows-path-to-suicide-prevention-in-covid-recovery.html (accessed on 24 August 2021).
9. Australian Institute of Health and Welfare. Ambulance Attendances: Suicidal and Self-Harm Behaviours. Available online: https://www.aihw.gov.au/suicide-self-harm-monitoring/data/ambulance-attendances/ambulance-attendances-for-suicidal-behaviours (accessed on 20 July 2021).
10. Australian Institute of Health and Welfare. Australia's Youth. Available online: https://www.aihw.gov.au/reports/children-youth/australias-youth/contents/about (accessed on 28 June 2021).
11. Biddle, N.; Gray, M. *Tracking Outcomes during the COVID-19 Pandemic (October 2020)—Reconvergence. COVID-19 Briefing Paper*; ANU Centre for Social Research and Methods: Canberra, Australia, 2020.
12. Melbourne Institute. *Coping with COVID-19: Rethinking Australia*; University of Melbourne: Melbourne, Australia, 2020.
13. Biddle, N.; Edwards, B.; Gary, M.; Sollis, K. *Hardship, Distress, and Resilience: The Initial Impacts of COVID-19 in Australia*; ANU Centre for Social Research and Methods: Canberra, Australia, 2020.
14. OECD Policy Responses to Coronavirus (COVID-19): Tackling the Mental Health Impact of the COVID-19 Crisis: An Integrated, Whole-of-Society Response. Available online: https://www.oecd.org/coronavirus/policy-responses/tackling-the-mental-health-impact-of-the-covid-19-crisis-an-integrated-whole-of-society-response-0ccafa0b/ (accessed on 21 September 2021).
15. Australian Institute of Health and Welfare. Mental Health Services in Australia: Overview of Mental Health Services in Australia. Available online: https://www.aihw.gov.au/reports/mental-health-services/mental-health-services-in-australia/report-contents/summary-of-mental-health-services-in-australia/overview-of-mental-health-services-in-australia (accessed on 22 September 2021).
16. National Mental Health Commission. *National Mental Health and Wellbeing Pandemic Response Plan*; Australian Government: Canberra, Australia, 2020.
17. Services Australia. Education Guide—Better Access to Mental Health Care for Eligible Health Professionals. Available online: https://www.servicesaustralia.gov.au/organisations/health-professionals/topics/education-guide-better-access-mental-health-care-eligible-health-professionals/35591 (accessed on 29 June 2021).
18. Australian Government Department of Health. Additional 10 Mental Health Sessions during COVID-19. Available online: https://www.health.gov.au/sites/default/files/documents/2020/10/additional-10-mbs-mental-health-sessions-during-covid-19-faqs-for-consumers-additional-10-mbs-mental-health-sessions-during-covid-19-faqs-for-consumers.pdf (accessed on 27 July 2021).
19. Australian Institute of Health and Welfare. Mental Health Services in Australia: Data Sources and Key Concepts, Pharmaceutical Benefits Scheme and Repatriation Pharmaceutical Benefits Scheme Data. Available online: https://www.aihw.gov.au/reports/mental-health-services/mental-health-services-in-australia/report-contents/mental-health-related-prescriptions/data-source-and-key-concepts (accessed on 22 September 2021).
20. Australian Government Department of Health. Coronavirus (COVID-19) at a Glance—25 April 2021. Available online: https://www.health.gov.au/resources/publications/coronavirus-covid-19-at-a-glance-21-april-2021 (accessed on 27 July 2021).
21. Australian Institute of Health and Welfare. Mental Health Services in Australia: Data Sources and Key Concepts, Medicare Benefits Schedule Data. Available online: https://www.aihw.gov.au/reports/mental-health-services/mental-health-services-in-australia/report-contents/medicare-subsidised-services/data-source-and-key-concepts (accessed on 22 September 2021).
22. Australian Government Services Australia. Medicare Item Reports. Available online: http://medicarestatistics.humanservices.gov.au/statistics/mbs_item.jsp (accessed on 22 September 2021).
23. WHO Collaborating Centre for Drug Statistics Methodology. Structure and Principles. Available online: https://www.whocc.no/atc/structure_and_principles/ (accessed on 22 September 2021).

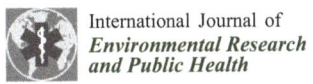

Review

Health Expenditure Data, Analysis and Policy Relevance in Australia, 1967 to 2020

John R. Goss

Health Research Institute, Faculty of Health, University of Canberra, Canberra 2617, Australia; john.goss@canberra.edu.au

Abstract: Since 1985, the Australian Institute of Health and Welfare (AIHW) has published 85 health expenditure publications. It has gradually extended the scope of these publications by extending the health accounts to detail expenditure by disease and age/sex, by State, Territory and remoteness and by Indigenous status. These enhanced health expenditure databases were then used to understand in detail the drivers of health expenditure. Understanding the drivers of health expenditure enables policy makers to understand where to intervene so as to maximise the health improvements that arise from health expenditure growth.

Keywords: health expenditure; health expenditure projections; disease expenditure; health expenditure policy

Citation: Goss, J.R. Health Expenditure Data, Analysis and Policy Relevance in Australia, 1967 to 2020. *Int. J. Environ. Res. Public Health* **2022**, *19*, 2143. https://doi.org/10.3390/ijerph19042143

Academic Editors: Richard Madden and Matthew Taylor

Received: 15 December 2021
Accepted: 9 February 2022
Published: 14 February 2022

Publisher's Note: MDPI stays neutral with regard to jurisdictional claims in published maps and institutional affiliations.

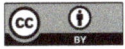

Copyright: © 2022 by the author. Licensee MDPI, Basel, Switzerland. This article is an open access article distributed under the terms and conditions of the Creative Commons Attribution (CC BY) license (https://creativecommons.org/licenses/by/4.0/).

1. History of Health Expenditure Data Collection and Publication in Australia

The first comprehensive set of health expenditure numbers for Australia was published by John Deeble in 1967 [1]. These estimates set the scene for the development work by Deeble and Scotton, leading to the introduction of universal health insurance in Australia in 1975 [2].

The first health expenditure publication by the Commonwealth Department of Health "Australian health expenditure 1974–75 to 1977–78: An analysis" was issued in 1980 [3]. This was followed by 3 updates in 1981, 1983 and 1985 [4–6].

The health expenditure collection and publication function was transferred to the Australian Institute of Health (AIH) when it was established as a separate Division within the Commonwealth Department of Health in 1985. The first health expenditure monograph published by the AIH was published in 1988 [7].

The author of this paper first became involved in health expenditure collection, analysis and publication at the AIH in 1986 and concluded his work on health expenditure at the Institute in 2010, so this paper reflects the views of an insider. The perspective of the author needs to be understood in interpreting the views expressed in this paper.

Since then, the AIH, or the Australian Institute of Health and Welfare (AIHW) as it became, has published 85 health expenditure publications [8]. Dissemination of information is a prime part of the mission of the AIHW, whereas the prime role of the Commonwealth Department of Health is policy advice and implementation and these functions tend to crowd out its information dissemination role. Additionally, because the Institute became an independent statutory authority of the Commonwealth Government in 1987, the analysis that accompanies the data is bolder and more independent than analyses from government health departments.

The Australian health expenditure accounts are mostly collated according to the rules and classifications of the System of Health Accounts [9]. Such classification systems have their inadequacies in that they have to classify expenditure into one category or another, so the multipurpose nature of most expenditure is not captured. However, these classification systems have the advantage that they classify expenditure fairly consistently across countries and across States and Territories within Australia.

Having a consistent set of definitions for health expenditure in Australia's Metadata Online Repository (METeOR) is a necessary first step in developing datasets which are consistent across jurisdictions, but much work needs to be carried out to encourage the Australian States and Territories and the Commonwealth Government to provide data according to these definitions.

2. Aboriginal and Torres Strait Islander Health Expenditure

Australia was the first country to comprehensively estimate how much was spent on health services for its Indigenous Aboriginal and Torres Strait Islander population. This was carried out in a report by Deeble, Mathers, Smith and Goss published in 1998 [10]. This report estimated that per person health expenditure from all sources for Indigenous people in 1995–1996 was 8% higher than for non-Indigenous people. As the health status of Indigenous people was so much worse, with a life expectancy gap of at least 12 years, it was clear that the 8% higher per person expenditure was not enough to address the much greater need for health services of Aboriginal and Torres Strait Islander people. Up until this publication, it was the popular view that large amounts were spent on health services for Indigenous people and a significant portion of this expenditure was wasted. After this publication, that view was no longer tenable. Spending was shown to be particularly low for Australian Government-funded medical benefits and pharmaceuticals. This report led the Commonwealth Department of Health to increase substantially its funding for Aboriginal and Torres Strait Islander health services both to start to address the identified deficit in funding of Indigenous health and because the report showed the States were funding a greater proportion of Indigenous health expenditure as compared to the Commonwealth Government.

The report also exposed deficiencies in the identification of Aboriginal and Strait Islander people in health data collections and helped lead to improvements in identification in these collections.

Indigenous health expenditure estimates have continued to be refined over the years [11], including estimates being made of Indigenous health expenditure by remoteness and by disease [12]. The ratio of Indigenous to non-Indigenous health funding per person has increased substantially from 1.08 in 1995–96 to 1.30 in 2015–16 [13].

2.1. Disease Expenditure Data

The first comprehensive disease expenditure data for Australia were published by the AIHW in 1998 for the reference year 1993–94 [14]. These were world leading data. Many countries had published data for expenditure for particular diseases, and particularly for the government-funded portion of that expenditure. However, no other country had published expenditure data for each disease, for government- and private-funded expenditure and for almost all areas of expenditure. This disease expenditure publications dissected expenditure by disease for 90% of recurrent expenditure in 1993–94. Disease expenditure data were published subsequently for 2000–01, 2004–05, 2015–16 and 2018–19 [15–18].

In 2018–19, musculoskeletal disorders accounted for 10.3% of recurrent health expenditure which could be allocated by disease, followed by cardiovascular disease at 8.7%. Cancer accounted for 8.6% of expenditure, mental illness 7.7% and injury 7.6%. Reproductive and maternal conditions accounted for 6.7% and oral disorders for 6.5%. It is noteworthy that while much of the discourse in health is about interventions that reduce mortality, that leading reasons for health expenditure include assisting mothers to give birth and the low mortality conditions of musculoskeletal disorders, mental illness and oral disorders.

The great strength of the disease expenditure analyses performed by the AIHW is that it is performed within the standard health expenditure framework. Many disease costing studies attempt to estimate the total social cost of a disease including indirect costs such as the loss of productivity due to a person dying from disease. The problem with this approach is that when the costs of all the different diseases are added up, the total number is many times total health expenditure. The AIHW approach allows the expenditure caused by a particular disease to be compared to actual real world health expenditure.

2.2. Public Health Expenditure

A detailed dissection of public health expenditure into 9 categories for each of the States and Territories and for the Commonwealth Government was produced in 2001 for the reference year 1998–99 [19]. These detailed data were published until the reference year 2008–09 [20], after which it ceased as the Commonwealth Department of Health stopped funding it. The nine categories of expenditure were immunisation (28% of public health expenditure in 2008–09), health promotion (19%), communicable disease control (12%), food standards and hygiene (2%), breast cancer and cervical screening (15%), and prevention of harmful drug use and public health research (7%). The per person public health expenditure was similar across the 6 States, but was 50% higher for the Australian Capital Territory) (ACT) and 300% higher for the Northern Territory (NT) in 2008–09. Over the 10 years for which these detailed data were published, the variation of State per person expenditure from the national mean State per person expenditure reduced by 50%.

Public health expenditure, as recorded in these reports, was $1014 million in 2000–01 [21]. In addition to this core public health expenditure, there was substantial expenditure on primary health care services and pharmaceuticals which reduced hypertension and cholesterol. This public health-related expenditure was $2140 million in 2000–01.

In total, core public health and public health-related expenditure came to $3154 million in 2000–01. Although this was only 5.9% of total recurrent health expenditure in 2000–01, it was responsible for a disproportionate proportion of the improvement in health that occurred around this period. So, for example, reductions in smoking, systolic blood pressure and cholesterol accounted for 74% of the male decline and 81% of the female decline in the coronary heart disease mortality rate in the period 1968–2000 [22].

3. Drivers of Health Expenditure Growth

Health expenditure grows every year, and usually at rates which are higher than other sectors in the economy. Health expenditure as a percentage of GDP has grown from 7.6% of GDP in 1978–79 to 10.0% of GDP in 2018–19 [23]. The question as to why health expenditure is growing at such a high rate is frequently asked. Following on from this, questions are asked as to whether the growth in health expenditure is sustainable and whether this increase in expenditure is achieving value for money.

To answer these questions, we must first understand the drivers of health expenditure. How much of health expenditure growth is due to the demographic factors of ageing and population growth? How much health expenditure growth is due to changing disease and risk factor levels? How much growth is due to the higher price of health goods and services relative to prices in the rest of the economy? Additionally, how much of health expenditure growth is due to higher rates of services provided per case of disease? Analysis of the drivers of health expenditure growth 50 years ago was very much in its infancy but as the years have gone by, decomposition analysis of health expenditure drivers has become more complete and sophisticated.

Table 1 below shows the decomposition of growth in 3 major areas of health expenditure for from 2000–01 to 2011–12 and from 2011–12 to 2018–19. The decomposition uses the Das Gupta decomposition method [24,25]. These three areas of hospital admitted patient services, medical services and pharmaceuticals together accounted for 55% of recurrent health expenditure in 2018–19. Health expenditure for these three areas grew in real terms at an average pace of 5.0% per year from 2000–01 to 2011–12 and at an average pace of 3.1% per year from 2011–12 to 2018–19. (Expenditure is calculated in real terms by deflating expenditure by the Gross National Expenditure (GNE) deflator. The GNE deflator is a good measure of general inflation in the economy as a whole and is the most appropriate deflator to use when comparing the value of money spent in the health sector as compared to money spent elsewhere.)

Table 1. Drivers of real health expenditure growth, from 2000–01 to 2011–12 and from 2011–12 to 2017–18.

Drivers of Real Health Expenditure Growth	2000–01 to 2011–12	2011–12 to 2017–18
Total real annual average growth	5.0%	3.1%
Demographic growth	**1.8%**	**1.7%** [1]
Population growth	1.1%	1.1%
Ageing	0.7	0.6
Non-demographic growth	**3.1%**	**1.4%** [2]
Excess health price inflation	0.34%	0.14%
Disease rate changes	−0.08%	0.07%
Growth in services per case of disease	2.8%	1.2%

Numbers in Table 1 calculated by author from [23]. [1] "Demographic growth" combines "Population growth" and "Ageing". [2] "Non-demographic growth" combines "Excess health price inflation", "Disease rate changes" and "Growth in services per case of disease".

The 5.0% annual growth from 2000–01 to 2011–12 can then be decomposed into the demographic component of 1.8% per year and the non-demographic component of 3.1% per year. The demographic component is then decomposed into the population growth component of 1.1% per year and the ageing component of 0.7%. The non-demographic component can be decomposed into three factors—excess health price inflation which adds 0.34% per year to real health expenditure growth and changing rates of disease which reduces health expenditure growth by 0.08% per year. (The projections section discusses more about this surprising result.) The residual component of health expenditure growth adds 2.8% per year. This component represents how much real health expenditure has increased due to more health goods and services being delivered per case of disease.

This increase in services per case of disease is the key parameter in determining whether an increase in health expenditure is value for money. One would normally expect to see an increase in health system attributable outcomes of at least 2.8% per year in order to justify an increase in services per case of disease of 2.8% per year. From 2003 to 2011, a measure of health outcomes—age-standardised Disability Adjusted Life Year (DALY) rates—declined by 1.1% per year. This is a strong indication that the rate of increase in health expenditure in this period was not value for money.

Further work needs to be carried out to ascertain whether there really was a decline in health productivity in this period, but disease expenditure data enable analysis to be performed as to whether increases in disease expenditure inputs result in commensurate disease improvements.

There was a significantly lower growth rate in real expenditure from 2011–12 to 2018–19 as compared to from 2000–01 to 2011–12 of only 3.1% per year.

Almost all of this lower growth is due to services delivered per case of disease growing at 1.2% per year as compared to the 2.8% per year rate of growth for this factor from 2000–01 to 2011–12.

In order to ensure that health expenditure grows at an optimal rate, it is primarily the growth in services per case of disease which must be controlled. This factor grows due to changes in treatment practices, changes in technology and changes in consumer preferences.

Some of the systems which control health expenditure growth, such as hospital casemix funding, have been unhelpful as they have allocated resources without understanding which growth is necessary and improves health, and which growth is wasteful and detracts from health. The Pharmaceutical Benefits Advisory Committee and the Medical Services Advisory Committee have followed a better way of restraining wasteful expenditure by evaluating whether new pharmaceuticals or new medical services are cost-effective.

Understanding growth in services per case of disease, and how this growth results in health outcome improvements, is another approach to fostering increases in expenditure which improve health.

4. Health Price Increases and General Inflation

Health prices generally increase faster than general inflation because the health sector is dominated by services, and the price of services in a growing economy goes up on average faster than the price of goods [26,27]. This amount by which health prices increase faster than general inflation is called 'excess health price inflation' and, as shown above, is a significant driver of health expenditure increases.

However, it is important to understand that excess health inflation is different for each health price index, and the extent of excess health inflation varies over time.

Table 2 shows excess health price inflation relative to the GNE deflator for health prices as a whole, and for hospital, medical, dental and pharmaceutical prices.

Table 2. Excess health price inflation relative to GNE deflator, annual average growth, from 2002–03 to 2018–19.

Excess Health Price Inflation	2002–03 to 2009–10	2009–10 to 2014–15	2014–15 to 2016–17	2016–17 to 2018–19	2002–03 to 2018–19
Total excess health price inflation	0.72%	−0.32%	0.86%	0.05%	0.33%
Excess hospital price inflation	0.99%	0.37%	0.63%	1.05%	0.76%
Excess medical price inflation	1.51%	−0.32%	−0.59%	−0.72%	0.39%
Excess dental price inflation	1.76%	−0.95%	−2.04%	−0.92%	0.09%
Excess pharmaceutical price inflation	−1.63%	−4.32%	11.28%	−5.29%	−1.43%

Numbers in Table 2 calculated by author from [23].

From 2002–03 to 2009–10, excess health price inflation for health prices as a whole was 0.72% per year. Excess hospital price inflation was 0.99% per year and excess medical price inflation was 1.51% per year. (The medical price deflator used here is the Medicare medical service fee charged deflator.) The Pharmaceutical Benefits Scheme (PBS) recorded a negative pharmaceutical excess price inflation of 1.63% per year during this period.

From 2009–10 to 2014–15, overall excess health price inflation was unusually negative at −0.32% per year. Although excess hospital price inflation was positive at 0.37% per year, excess medical, dental and pharmaceutical price inflation were all negative, leading to the overall negative result.

From 2009–10 to 2018–19, excess medical price inflation was almost always negative due to the government severely limiting increases in the benefits proscribed by the Medicare Benefits Schedule (MBS). The 11% annual average increase in excess pharmaceutical price inflation from 2014–15 to 2016–17 was due almost entirely to expensive Hepatitis C pharmaceuticals being added to the PBS.

5. Health Expenditure Projections

Projections for components of Australian health expenditure have been undertaken for many years in Australia, e.g., the Commonwealth Intergenerational Reports project Commonwealth health expenditure 40 years into the future [28]. However, more sophisticated projections only became possible when burden of disease analyses became available. Burden of disease analyses estimate the overall impact of disease by estimating the impact of disease in reducing life expectancy and its impact in increasing illness and reducing functioning. The overall burden of disease is measured using a metric called the Disability Adjusted Life Year (DALY). The DALY consists of the premature mortality component called the Years of Life Lost (Years of Life Lost), and healthy life years lost due to illness and reduced functioning called the Years of Life lost due to Disability (YLD). The burden of disease analyses estimate not just the burden imposed by each disease, but also the prevalence, incidence, severity and sequelae of disease, and the risk factors that increase the risk of disease [29].

The first projection of Australian health expenditure that took into account disease projections was a report for the United Nations World Economic and Social Survey 2007 by Vos, Goss, Begg and Mann [30].

Then, in 2009, Goss reworked this projection for the National Health and Hospitals Reform Commission [31]. This study produced some surprising results.

First, this study estimated that changing disease rates over the 30 years 2002–03 to 2032–33 were expected to lead to a net reduction in health expenditure of $2.3 billion. Although expected increases in the disease rates for diabetes and other diseases would lead to increased expenditure of $4.7 billion, expected decreases in expenditure on heart disease, cancer and other diseases would lead to savings of $7.4 billion, leading to net savings of $2.3 billion.

Second, ageing was not the main driver of health expenditure that many people expected. Of the projected increase in health and residential aged care expenditure of $161 billion, only $38 billion (23%) was due to ageing.

Third, the biggest factor expected to drive health expenditure increases was the growth in the amount of health services provided per case of disease. This factor was expected to grow by $81 billion in the 20 years to 2032–2033, which was 50% of the overall increase. The growth of this factor is mostly under the control of the health system (in contrast to the other drivers of health expenditure which are mostly not). For each case of presenting disease, providers mostly have the power to choose over time to provide more (or less) services per case of disease, and consumers also have some power to demand more (or less) services per case of disease.

This projection model was used to inform recommendations to the Commonwealth Government by the National Health and Hospitals Reform Commission in areas such as the impact of a reduction in smoking, an increase in aged care places, the improved treatment of diabetes and a reduced rate of increase in obesity rates [32].

6. Conclusions: Impact of Health Expenditure Data and Analysis on Health Policy in Australia, 1967 to 2020

Health expenditure data have been influential in shaping debates about health policy in Australia and in shaping health policy itself.

The health expenditure data that John Deeble collected and analysed in the 1960s were critical in shaping the policy recommendations from Deeble and Scotton that were crucial in the establishment of Medibank in 1975.

Information about what was actually spent on health services for Aboriginal and Torres Strait Islander people changed the policy debate from one focussed on reducing 'waste' in spending on health services for Aboriginal and Torres Strait Islander people to addressing major unmet needs in expenditure on these services.

For decades, health expenditure as a proportion of GDP has been a marker of the debate as to whether too much or too little was being spent on health services in Australia. However, only when there is a detailed understanding of the drivers of health expenditure as a proportion of GDP is it possible to have an informed debate as to how much should be spent on health and where it should be spent. This understanding of what drives health expenditure depends on a detailed understanding of where the money is spent—how much is spent by hospitals, medical practices, pharmacies, etc., how much is spent by governments, health insurance funds and individuals, how much is spent for each age/sex group, how much is spent for the prevention and treatment of each disease, how much is spent for different socioeconomic groups, for Aboriginal and Torres Strait Islanders and for people living in different regions of Australia. In the last 50 years, we have developed our understanding of the details of what is spent on health and for whom and for what purpose, so that now, when we link this detailed expenditure information to the health outcomes it engenders, we are able to more wisely allocate our health expenditure so as to achieve higher-quality health care for all.

Funding: This research received no external funding.

Institutional Review Board Statement: Not applicable.

Informed Consent Statement: Not applicable.

Data Availability Statement: All data used are referenced in References.

Acknowledgments: The support of the Academic Editor of this Special Issue—Richard Madden—is gratefully acknowledged.

Conflicts of Interest: The author declares no conflict of interest at this point of time, but readers should be aware that the author was centrally involved in the collection, analysis and publication of health expenditure data at the Australian Institute of Health and Welfare from 1986 to 2010.

References

1. Deeble, J.S. The costs and sources of finance of Australian health services. *Econ. Rec.* **1967**, *43*, 518–543. [CrossRef]
2. Scotton, R.B.; Macdonald, C.R. *The Making of Medibank*; School of Health Services Management, University of NSW: Sydney, Australia, 1993.
3. Commonwealth Department of Health. *Australian Health Expenditure 1974–75 to 1977–78: An Analysis*; AGPS: Canberra, Australia, 1980.
4. Commonwealth Department of Health. *Australian Health Expenditure 1974–75 to 1978–79: An Analysis*; AGPS: Canberra, Australia, 1981.
5. Commonwealth Department of Health. *Australian Health Expenditure 1975–76 to 1979–80: An Analysis*; AGPS: Canberra, Australia, 1983.
6. Commonwealth Department of Health. *Australian Health Expenditure 1979–80 to 1981–82*; Australian Institute of Health (AIH): Canberra, Australia, 1985.
7. Goss, J.R.; Harvey, R.; Greenhill, D. *Australian Health Expenditure 1970–71 to 1984–85*; AIHW: Canberra, Australia, 1988.
8. Australian Institute of Health and Welfare Expenditure Publications. Available online: https://www.aihw.gov.au/reports-data/health-welfare-overview/health-welfare-expenditure/reports (accessed on 12 January 2022).
9. OECD; Eurostat; World Health Organization. *A System of Health Accounts 2011, Revised ed.*; OECD Publishing: Paris, France, 2017.
10. Deeble, J.; Mathers, C.; Smith, J.; Goss, J. *Expenditures on Health Services for Aboriginal and Torres Strait Islander People*; Public Affairs, Parliamentary and Access Branch, Commonwealth Department of Health and Family Services: Canberra, Australia, 1998.
11. Deeble, J.; Shelton Agar, J.; Goss, J. *Expenditures on Health for Aboriginal and Torres Strait Islander Peoples 2004–05*; AIHW: Canberra, Australia, 2008.
12. Australian Institute of Health and Welfare. *Expenditure on Health for Aboriginal and Torres Strait Islander People 2010–11: An Analysis by Remoteness and Disease*; AIHW: Canberra, Australia, 2013.
13. Australian Institute of Health and Welfare. *Aboriginal and Torres Strait Islander Health Performance Framework 2020 Summary Report*; AIHW: Canberra, Australia, 2020.
14. Mathers, C.; Penm, R.; Carter, R.; Stevenson, C. *Health System Costs of Diseases and Injury in Australia 1993–94*; AIHW: Canberra, Australia, 1998.
15. Australian Institute of Health and Welfare. *Health System Expenditure on Disease and Injury in Australia 2000–01*; AIHW: Canberra, Australia, 2005.
16. Australian Institute of Health and Welfare. *Health System Expenditure on Disease and Injury in Australia 2004–05*; AIHW: Canberra, Australia, 2010.
17. Australian Institute of Health and Welfare. *Disease Expenditure in Australia 2015–16*; AIHW: Canberra, Australia, 2021.
18. Australian Institute of Health and Welfare. *Disease Expenditure in Australia 2018–19*; AIHW: Canberra, Australia, 2020.
19. Australian Institute of Health and Welfare. *National Public Health Expenditure Report 1998–99*; AIHW: Canberra, Australia, 2001.
20. Australian Institute of Health and Welfare. *Public Health Expenditure In Australia 2008–09*; AIHW: Canberra, Australia, 2011.
21. Australian Institute of Health and Welfare. *National Public Health Expenditure Report 2000–01*; AIHW: Canberra, Australia, 2002.
22. Taylor, R.; Dobson, A.; Mirsaei, M. Contribution of changes in risk factors to the decline of coronary heart disease mortality in Australia over three decades. *Eur. J. Cardiovasc. Prev. Rehabil.* **2006**, *13*, 760–768. [CrossRef] [PubMed]
23. Australian Institute of Health and Welfare. *Health Expenditure Database*; AIHW: Canberra, Australia, 2021.
24. Das Gupta, P. Current Population Reports. In *Standardization and Decomposition of Rates: A User's Manual*; Bureau of the Census: Washington, DC, USA, 1993.
25. Zhai, T.; Goss, J.; Li, J. Main drivers of health expenditure growth in China: A decomposition analysis. *BMC Health Serv. Res.* **2017**, *17*, 185. [CrossRef] [PubMed]
26. Hartwig, J. Can Baumol's model of unbalanced growth contribute to explaining the secular rise in health care expenditure? An alternative test. *Appl. Econ.* **2011**, *43*, 173–184. [CrossRef]
27. Baumol, W.J. *Baumol's Cost Disease: The Arts and Other Victims*; Edward Elgar: Aldershot, UK, 1997.
28. The Treasury. *2021 Intergenerational Report Australia over the Next 40 Years*; Commonwealth of Australia: Canberra, Australia, 2021.

29. Mathers, C.; Vos, T.; Stevenson, C. *The Burden of Disease and Injury in Australia*; Australian Institute of Health and Welfare: Canberra, Australia, 1999.
30. Begg, S.; Vos, T.; Goss, J.; Mann, N. An alternative approach to projecting health expenditure in Australia. *Aust. Health Rev.* **2008**, *32*, 148–155. [CrossRef] [PubMed]
31. Goss, J. *Projection of Australian Health Care Expenditure by Disease 2003 to 2033*; AIHW: Canberra, Australia, 2008.
32. Goss, J. *Estimating the Impact of Selected National Health and Hospitals Reform Commission (NHHRC) Reforms on Health Care Expenditure, 2003 to 2033*; AIHW: Canberra, Australia, 2009.

MDPI
St. Alban-Anlage 66
4052 Basel
Switzerland
Tel. +41 61 683 77 34
Fax +41 61 302 89 18
www.mdpi.com

International Journal of Environmental Research and Public Health Editorial Office
E-mail: ijerph@mdpi.com
www.mdpi.com/journal/ijerph

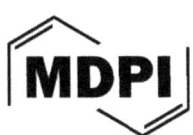